MIRACLES
and
MAYHEM
in the ER

Unbelievably True Stories from an
Emergency Room Doctor

elevate

Elevate, USA

Published in Boise, Idaho by Elevate
www.elevatepub.com

This book may be purchased in bulk for educational, business, organizational,
or promotional use.

For information please email info@russell-media.com.

ISBN (print): 978-1-937498-22-1
ISBN (e-book): 978-1-937498-23-8

Printed in the United States of America

AUTHOR'S NOTE

◫ ◫ ◫

The patients and events in this book are factual. These events occurred during my residency and shortly after. See afterword for full disclosure. Emergency medicine is stranger than fiction.

—BRENT RUSSELL, MD
Emergency Physician

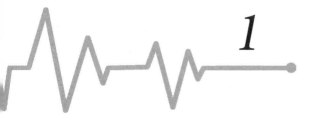

1

"Your next patient is Cannibal Cullison. He's eager to feed. Don't let his teeth near your face." A gray-haired nurse—ex-military—dourly handed me the chart.

I asked, "What?"

She tilted her chin forward, snapped her teeth shut twice, and walked away with ramrod straight posture. I guessed she was trying to spook the new resident. I played it cool, although I probably blanched.

The Veterans Administration Hospital is affiliated with the Oregon Medical School and the Emergency Medicine Residency. I was a new resident in the program and I was assigned to the VA. VA patients are ex-military, a fact I had vaguely known for a long time but was vividly confirmed by the number of amputated patients I saw in the halls. Most are grateful for their care, but some feel betrayed—by their government, and by society.

Mr. Cullison had come to the ER with shortness of breath. I flipped through his bulky chart; he had severe heart disease, suffering multiple heart attacks in his fifty-one years, but these did not cause his heart of darkness.

He had severe congestive heart failure, causing a miserable and likely abbreviated existence. In plain terms, he could not walk from the parking lot to the grocery without stopping to rest. Mr. Cullison had lost two thirds of his heart; the remnant of which struggled like a tired old Wal-Mart greeter laboring long after he ached to retire.

His doctors had been unable to balance the fluids in his body. This heart condition coupled with his poor circulation would cause fluid to build up in his body. Diuretics were used to attempt fluid balance. Too much fluid not only caused his legs to swell like tree trunks, but the excess fluid also gathered in his lungs, causing a suffocating sensation. Too little fluid brought dehydration that caused injury to his kidneys due to poor perfusion of blood. The dehydration also led him to feel parched—a dusty soul wandering the desert.

I felt mounting unease as I flipped through his chart. I read about his psychiatric problems: post-traumatic stress disorder (PTSD) and rage issues. He had been to prison twice, the first time for beating a neighbor with a tire iron over a dispute involving dog feces in his yard. Later, he had completely bitten off a man's top lip in a bar fight. He then chewed the lip and swallowed it, leaving nothing to be reattached. Mr. Cullison had been in the ER for injuries he sustained in that fight, and returned to prison.

After reviewing the chart, I remembered the nurse's snapping teeth and I was rattled. The man sounded volatile. Aggressive patients made me nervous, especially since I was still green.

I would treat him with respect like any other patient, but I would not be intimidated—I hoped. As I headed across the large room, with fifteen beds lining three walls in a U shape, I steeled myself. I became self-consciously aware of my walking, as if I needed to think about taking each next step forward. I sensed the ill patients looking at me. I felt how hard the yellowish linoleum was under my shoes. The antiseptic smell of the ER mixed with a faint human odor, a nauseating odor of sickness. I took in the bland tan walls cluttered with wires, monitors, and charts. The entire place felt unwelcome and unnatural.

I walked to Mr. Cullison's bedside. He was bald and thick. His hospital gown was open, exposing his broad, hairy back. He sat on the side of his bed, wheezing into an oxygen mask.

I said, "Hello, Mr. Cullison. I'm Brent Russell, one of the emergency medicine residents." I extended my hand and he ignored it, leaving me holding the awkward pose. I lowered my hand, feeling even more apprehensive.

He stopped panting, pulled off the oxygen mask, and muttered, "Listen, kid, you people have to do something. I haven't been able to sleep for days. I'm huffing and puffing all night. If I fall asleep, I wake up feeling like I'm drowning." With a wheeze, he replaced the oxygen mask and breathed heavily, his nostrils flaring—a glint of mortal fear.

"We'll do everything we can. I'm not sure you'll be well enough to go home today."

Off came the mask again. "I'm so sick of this. This cursed hospital will tweak my meds and then schedule a recheck in a month," he said sarcastically. "I feel like I'm chained underwater, constantly struggling to keep my nose above the surface. I was shot in 'Nam and this is the thanks I get? Fifteen minutes, once a month, by a jellybean med student?"

I said, "I'm sorry you feel you've been getting the run around."

He continued savagely, "In service of my country, I've seen some things. I saw my best friend have both arms blown off by a booby trap." He paused and studied my face, looking for I don't know what. Compassion? Comprehension of what he'd been through? Shock?

He broke off his stare and added, "Ralph's wife still calls me on their wedding anniversary to hear how he said he loved her before he took his last swallow of air. I've spent thirty years having nightmares." He seemed to be telling me his story because he had no one else to tell, or because he spent every day reliving it.

"I've never been able to hold a job—or hold a wife—due to my anger. The last thing I held with love was Ralph's armless body."

I flinched at the image.

He took a deep breath and fixated on my face again. "I have righteous anger, doc, righteous anger."

I averted my eyes from his bitter glare and tried to change the subject. "How far can you walk across the room without getting short of breath? Any recent chest pain?" He seemed annoyed, but I wanted to move on as quickly as possible.

He answered my questions, and I proceeded to perform a physical exam. When I listened to his lungs with my stethoscope, I heard a crackly, Velcro-like sound, indicating fluid instead of air. His swollen lower legs dented when I pushed with a finger, indicating fluid retention. His flabby heart was failing to pump the fluid out.

I went to the doctor's workroom to order blood work, an EKG, a chest X-ray, and medicines. I was relieved to be out of his oppressive presence.

He was right; congestive heart failure is like drowning in your own body—the skin becomes a bloated water balloon.

As I had learned in med school, the coronary arteries are small blood vessels that supply the heart muscle with blood. Cholesterol plaques build up and narrow the vessels. This restricts blood flow, causing angina, or chest pain. A heart attack is usually caused by rupture of a plaque, forming a blood clot and blocking blood flow. This disruption will cause the heart muscle downstream to die. The heart muscle can be spared if the clot dissolves, is removed, or is bypassed.

The clot can be removed by heart catheterization, a procedure performed by a cardiologist. The doctor feeds a catheter into a vein in the groin and up into the coronary arteries. A small balloon is

MIRACLES and MAYHEM in the ER

inflated to destroy the clot and reopen the blockage. A rigid tube, a stent, may be placed to keep the blockage open.

Clot-busting drugs are used when a cardiologist is not available. Clot-busting drugs destroy all blood clots in the body and can occasionally lead to devastating bleeding.

A blockage may be bypassed with open-heart surgery, or coronary artery bypass grafting. During this operation, a cardiac surgeon takes a vein from the patient's leg and sews it on both sides of a coronary artery, allowing blood to flow around the blockage.

None of these methods are foolproof because heart disease inevitably causes damage. Mr. Cullison's dark heart was testament to the unending destruction it causes.

I was attending another patient, but I could see Mr. Cullison from across the room; he looked agitated and restless. At one point he got out of bed and walked stiffly across the room. He took short shuffling steps and held his chin upward.

The gray-haired nurse whispered, "The Tin Man needs a new heart."

His movements did look sort of mechanical. Finally, he ended his walk by the nurses' station, where he began reading postings on a bulletin board.

The secretary, wearing thick makeup, sighed loudly, "May I help you?"

He said, "No, just mind your own business."

She retorted, "Sir, you need to go back to your bed, please. Now." She sharply pointed her fire red fingernail toward his bed.

He leaned down over the high counter, muttering through grinding teeth, "You have no idea who you're dealing with."

She didn't hesitate. She called loudly, "Security, please help Mr. Cullison back to his bed." Jason, the portly security guard, walked over and gently put his hand on the older man's arm, "Let's go, sir. Back to your bed."

Mr. Cullison jerked his arm away and spun to face the guard. Both hands became fists. He looked like he wanted to murder, maybe even cannibalize, his latest antagonist.

Smelling trouble, I walked over to attempt to calm him, but I could feel my palms sweating.

He stared menacingly at the security guard. Measuring the depth of the man's hostility, Jason took a step back and asked the secretary, "Can you call for backup?"

Mr. Cullison snarled, "Chump. Why do you need backup, fatso?"

With a semblance of military precision, he turned and walked back to his bed, panting. He seemed satisfied that he had stood his ground. I was relieved that a potentially volatile situation had been avoided.

I made the rounds with a few other patients— one with a sore throat, another with a diabetic foot ulcer, and a migraine headache sufferer. I saw an elderly World War II vet with pneumonia who needed to be admitted.

I checked my diagnosis of each patient with the attending physician. She listened to the five residents working in the ER that day about their patients' histories. She asked pertinent questions: "Does he have high blood pressure?" If we did not know the answer, she would instruct us to find out. She asked what medications we wanted to order, our treatment plan, and general medical questions. She had two roles: teaching and supervising. She attended most patients in a cursory manner, unless it was a complicated case or the resident was unsure.

A few minutes later, I realized the debacle was not over. From a distance Mr. Cullison was trying to goad Jason. He relentlessly glared at the security guard, and Jason ignored him. The veteran had emerged from the horrors of combat with a not uncommon result of PTSD. He was always looking for a fight.

The nurse had noticed, too. "Mr. Cullison is eyeballing Jason like a freaky-deeky psychopath," she warned me. "When are you going to get him out of the ER? I don't want him to go Hannibal Lecter."

That reminded me. "I have his labs and X-rays back. I'll talk with him after I review everything."

His chest x-ray showed pulmonary edema, fluid in his lungs. I ordered that he be assigned to a bed on the cardiac floor. He wanted to stay in the hospital, and he needed to stay. It is always much easier when the patient's desires and medical needs align, and, in his case, I was particularly glad they did. I did not want to fight with Mr. Cullison about his course of treatment.

I went to speak with him about his upcoming stay with us. All the while he stared at Jason—a slow burn—as he answered my questions.

"Is your shortness of breath better?"

"No."

"We should admit you to the hospital for a few days." I hoped this prospect would make him happy.

He turned to zero in on me. The crooked-toothed snarl and hooded brow made him looked like an animal—a sickly, rabid pit bull. "What makes you so sure, Doc? Because I can't walk far enough for you to discharge me?"

Mr. Cullison returned his granite stare to Jason. The VA Emergency Room often had angry patients, but he was a time bomb ready to explode. I was ready to get him out of the ER. The entire interaction was disquieting.

He would have to wait while a bed was prepared for him, and he was not a man to be kept waiting. A few minutes later, he pulled off his oxygen and marched to the nursing station. His eyes expanded, his veins protruded, and spittle flew from his mouth as he barked at the secretary, "Do you know what the Ho Chi Minh Offensive was?

Do you have any idea?"

"What?" she replied, startled. "Sir, you need to settle down." She pointed at his bed again.

He hissed, "You have no idea what we did for you and your country. You're an ungrateful, treasonous woman!"

He had crossed a line. Jason walked over and firmly gripped Mr. Cullison's left arm. When the Vietnam vet swung his right, Jason blocked the punch, pivoted around, and wrapped up Mr. Cullison with both arms from behind. As the older man vigorously struggled to be let go, Jason called for help.

I rushed toward them, my adrenaline surging. Mr. Cullison cursed and writhed desperately; he would hurt Jason if he got a chance. I grabbed a madly kicking leg and we knocked him to the ground in a semi-controlled manner.

Watch those teeth.

More help rushed into the ward. In short order, we had someone holding down each appendage. He snarled, "Jason Sampson, I'm going to kill you! I see your name badge. I will kill you. I'm not making a threat. I'm stating a fact."

We ignored his raving. A few nurses rolled his bed over.

But Mr. Cullison wouldn't stop. "I will kill you. You won't see it coming. You'll walk out of your house and I'll be in the bushes. You won't even see me as I sink a bullet into your skull. Or, you'll be walking to your car as I step out of an alley. Blam!"

He kept struggling, even though he was helplessly pinned down. "I'm very patient," he growled. "Our beloved country taught me to kill. You'll get up to go to the bathroom in the middle of the night and I'll be in your hallway. Crack! Brains splattered, as your wife screams and cries pitiful tears."

That idea made his eyes gleam. "I don't care, I'm dying anyway. It doesn't matter if I get caught. I have a very short time to live and my dying wish is to see you dead. To kill you with my own hands, Jason Sampson. To free your soul from that blubbery body so it can slither off to where it belongs." All of us were looking at each other uneasily, but he wouldn't shut up. "It may be next week and it may be in a few months, but I swear on Ralph's grave that I will kill you. You better sleep with one eye open."

Jason tried to look unfazed, but sweat was beading furiously on his forehead.

I snuck my hand up and removed my nametag.

Mr. Cullison stopped struggling, but he continued to taunt Jason as we lifted him onto the bed. Security personnel tied his hands and feet to the hospital bed with soft restraints.

The security guards remained by his bed. Mr. Cullison was laboring mightily to breathe; the fight had taken a toll. Watching those teeth, I put his oxygen mask back on.

A few minutes later, after my heartbeat had returned to a semblance of normalcy, I talked with my attending doctor about the best course of action. He needed to be admitted for his congestive heart failure, but he was a psychiatric case. In the end, we decided we would admit him to the cardiac floor with a constant security watch until he was medically stable. Then he would be placed in the psych ward.

The plan left me worried for Jason. What happened after Mr. Cullison spent a few days in the hospital and a few days on the psych ward? The police would probably cite him for threats, but in a few weeks' time he would be out on the loose.

⊡   ⊡   ⊡

Images of his rage-contorted face continued to haunt me. What had he seen that could have left him so violently unsettled? Had the death of his best friend been, as a psychologist would call it, the precipitating event that spawned a lifetime's struggle to maintain a hold on his sanity?

I was born during the Vietnam War. As a boy, I thought of soldiers as heroes who protected our country. With a child's self-absorption I equated their acts of derring-do with my own games of army in the woods by our house. I innocently asked my neighbor, a Vietnam vet, "Did you ever shoot anyone?" To my surprise, he did not answer, but his face grew stormy. I had the first inklings that war might be more serious than I imagined, but still I wanted to find out for sure. Another time, I asked him to tell me stories about the war, and he, uncharacteristically, became quiet and sullen. He said he couldn't talk about it.

I had a similar experience with my uncle, a gentle man with an easy laugh who fought in World War II. The greatest generation did not hesitate to answer the call of their country. During the war, I would learn, he was forced to crush wounded Germans, some of them civilians, under the treads of his tank. The description that stuck with me forever after was "skulls splattering like dropped watermelons."

As I grew older, my proximity to war would grow closer. Fred, the son of an African-American preacher in Mississippi, was one of the best friends I've ever had, and an exceptional person. His friendly, funny demeanor belied the fact that he could knock your football helmet sideways. We developed a unique friendship; we were from separate worlds in the Deep South, the first generation that attended integrated schools.

We were a rap duo, the B-Boys, and we performed at our school and other local venues. We spent countless hours writing songs, learning to scratch records, and making music. We even recorded an album in a studio. A few times we rapped and I was the only white person in the room.

My two best friends from high school joined the military: Steve went to the Air Force Academy and is currently the Commander of SEAL Team Three. Fred joined the Army and was stationed in Germany. After my sophomore year, I traveled to Europe to see Fred. He and I spent the summer traveling the continent, just the two of us. I was glad we could remain close as we got older.

The following year, Saddam invaded Kuwait and the first Iraq War erupted. The taped conversations brought Fred's fears of a war half a world away into my dorm room. On one tape he said, "If it's God's will for me to die over there, know that I love you. I've made you a recipient of my life insurance. That way you'll know if I die and maybe I can help you pay for med school." My eyes filled with tears. I couldn't imagine Fred getting killed.

I was alone in my fears. None of my college friends or family knew anyone going to war. I did not want to tell Fred I was scared, or that I disagreed with the war. I disagreed because whatever was going on there was not worth my friend's life.

Fred was not killed, but he did not emerge unscathed. Months later he would describe the missiles soaring overhead, wondering if they carried payloads of blistering, slow death, since Saddam had used chemical warfare on thousands of his own countrymen. After the invasion of Iraq began, Fred would pass burnt bodies, the skulls laughing like charred clowns. Some corpses were burnt in bizarre positions—such as a man standing by his vehicle, his hand still holding the door handle.

I could understand the effects of war intellectually. As part of my training, I learned that in war, the primitive part of the brain is unleashed. Freud called it the Id—the primal urges that prompt rage and fear, the flight or fight part of the brain. Biologists call it the reptilian brain—the deep brainstem structures that humans share with lizards and serpents; the selfish, creepy crawly part of the mind where our most basic needs and desires nest—food, sex, and violence. Just as being exposed to sex too young can cause a perverted expansion of the Id—pedophilia can create sex addicts—war opens a door that is hard to close. Normally kept in check by conscience and reason, war empowers the Id. When the Id is fed, it grows. Like a monster within, the Id can overpower and rule the conscience.

The marrow of the psyche is split open and mixed with mayhem and raw fear. The sight of a man's brain dripping down a wall leaves a searing image in the memory. If the brain is that of your friend, or spilled by your bullet, the memory can seem more vivid than current reality. That is what I suspect happened to Mr. Cullison.

Fred changed in a different way. He wasn't fearful, dissatisfied, or filled with hate, but upon his return, he seemed to have aged decades. He smiled less and often seemed lost in thought. He told me the civilian world seemed strange, like he was a visitor, or an alien. He had visited a harsher world and was still trying to find his way back.

The horrific effects of war have parallels to emergency medical training. Fear is fear, and adrenaline sears memories whether the bodies are viewed on the battlefield or rolling off an ambulance gurney. I saw my intern friends evolve in response to the mangled bodies they had to heal, and I felt myself do the same. I had thoughts and experiences that were beyond anything I had faced before. I became a first-hand witness to gore and mayhem, people ripped and torn open in all sorts of stomach-curdling ways. I saw mothers crying for dead babies, and babies crying for dead mommies. I tried to save them all and sometimes I would fail.

The victims of assault are often the worst. One chilling episode that will never leave me was a patient who shot himself in the head. He lived, but the bullet blew out his eyes. He came to the ER blinded, pleading with us to let him die. For weeks afterward the disturbing images would rear up at me unexpectedly. I found myself waking up in the middle of the night.

More often, medical trainees can be likened to frogs in slowly boiling water. We see sickness and death constantly, and if we are not careful, the doctor we had hoped to become will burn out. Out of necessity we create shells that protect and isolate us; sometimes it hurts too much to repeatedly feel another's pain. We laugh at things that are not funny. We discuss people in a dehumanized, detached way.

The difference between medicine and war, of course, is that we are trying to save lives, and soldiers are trained to kill. We are not fighting a hungry Id, bent on conquest and destruction. Our emotional wounds can receive the salve of our ability to heal.

But for Mr. Cullison, both his heart and his mind were ruined. The war had changed him into a beast that was barely human. Our country sent him to fight a proxy war against communism in a small country halfway around the world. The pain of war stuck to his soul like flaming napalm. The bomb that blew off Ralph's arms destroyed Mr. Cullison as well—only he had to stay aboveground, like a wraith wandering the world of the living. At least until that night when he unleashed mayhem in the emergency ward.

◻ ◻ ◻

I paged the internal medicine resident, and he responded crisply: "Dr. Brad McCoy, I was paged?"

"I have a patient with severe congestive heart failure who needs to be admitted." I outlined his medical history and current problems.

"Why can't you just increase his diuretics and send him home? Isn't he always like this?"

"This guy is sick," I told him. "His oxygen levels are in the mid eighties even on high-flow oxygen. Like I said, his chest X-ray looks terrible."

"Well, if he's that bad, he should go to the Intensive Care Unit. He sounds too sick to manage on the floor."

I was getting annoyed. "I don't think he needs the ICU now. But he does need to be admitted."

"I guess so, but if he's that sick, we're just going to transfer him to the ICU."

"He also had an altercation with one of our security guards. We had to take him down, and he's in restraints. He has rage issues."

"What? We can't have someone like that on our service! He needs to go to the psychiatric service! You should've told me that earlier!"

I tried to remain calm as I pointed out the obvious. "I'd be glad to call a psychiatric consult, but he can't be admitted on the psychiatric floor. They don't even have oxygen." I felt like saying, "Listen lazybones, we wrestled this flesh-eater to the ground and barely avoided being bitten. Just take the admission."

He said, "This is a terrible plan!"

"He's a difficult patient. Do you have a better idea?"

His voice was shrill, "I refuse this admission!"

My temper flared at last. "You can't refuse the admission."

"This is ludicrous!"

"If I haven't heard from you in twenty minutes, I'll send him to the floor," I informed him, and banged the phone down.

I sat for a minute to collect myself. Some residents are skilled at arguing about almost every admission. A new patient means more work for them—work they are not paid for. The first-year interns sometimes have to call third-year residents, who can volley back with their advanced knowledge: "Call me back when you've completed the work up and know the patient's most recent thyroid levels and their last echo report." This dynamic dissolves after residency. Non-resident physicians are not as overworked and they are paid for any additional work.

I was in the bathroom, splashing cold water on my face, when I heard an overhead page: "Dr. Russell, please come to room four immediately."

That was Mr. Cullison's room. My heart banged, I assumed he was raising a ruckus again.

I rushed in and was surprised to see Mr. Cullison limp and gray—not breathing. The nurses were trying to revive him.

I asked, "What happened?"

A nurse said, "The alarms sounded. He's in V fib!"

My eyes shot to the cardiac monitor: it showed the graph of ventricular fibrillation—a fatal heart rhythm. The heart was quivering instead of beating. V fib is a major cause of death in patients with congestive heart failure.

Life had drained from his eyes.

As I was trained, I struck his chest with my fist. This occasionally works to jolt the heart back into a normal rhythm. The fist can deliver about ten joules of power. It usually worked on *M*A*S*H*, but it did not work for me.

A nurse wheeled in the defibrillator. I grasped the paddles and pressed them to his chest. "Charge to two hundred joules. All clear?"

Shock.

Mr. Cullison's body jolted.

Nothing.

"Charge to three hundred."

Shock.

The cardiac monitor continued to show the chaotic vibration of V fib.

I rushed to the head of the bed, intubated him with a breathing tube, and we started chest compressions. We gave him resuscitation drugs: epinephrine, lidocaine.

We shocked him again and again.

Patients with severe congestive heart failure don't typically respond to resuscitation; they are like cancer patients. When their heart stops, that is usually the end. Game over. Lights out.

After forty-five minutes of resuscitation, we declared him dead. In the course of a few hours I had seen Mr. Cullison's face transform from fearful panic to a rabid pit bull to hate-filled chaos to a lifeless cold visage.

As I looked at his still form, I thought about my role and wondered if I could have done anything different. As a new resident, I did not have confidence in my abilities, and I often second-guessed my choices. To be confident at that stage of my training would be foolish, as I had been told over and over again.

I might have been able to diffuse Mr. Cullison's anger by getting a different security guard, but he probably would have hated any guard.

I thought the medical treatment was optimal. I might have discovered he was having a heart attack if I asked about chest pain after the altercation, but he did not volunteer the information, and I had asked about chest pain during the initial interview.

Still, I felt uneasy about his demise occurring under my care. The timing of his death was peculiar: why did he die less than an hour after threatening Jason? My supposition is that all along he was hanging on by a thread. His heart barely managed to get him to his mailbox, much less to take on six people. He overtaxed his very frail heart.

I covered Mr. Cullison with a sheet. I hoped he was finally at peace.

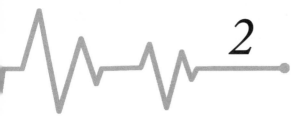

Looking back, I see fate had sealed my turbulent destiny. I really had no choice—emergency medicine chose me. From an early age, I wanted to be a doctor, although I spent a few years yearning to be one of the Dukes of Hazzard, running from the law. My two brothers and I played Bo, Luke, and Cooter on our Tennessee farm. Later, I ran from the cops more than once.

My sweet mother thought I would become a taxidermist, a doctor, or—Please, Lord. No!—a mortician because I dissected dead animals. A recently deceased possum was a prime patient for surgery. "Look mom, this part has green stuff inside."

I doubt any mamas long for their babies to be morticians. "Hello, Mother. I just drained the bile and washed out the intestines. Let's grab lunch before I remove her eyeballs."

I grew up in the heart of the Smoky Mountains, mostly outdoors. My parents encouraged imagination and exercise, exorcizing the television when I was a child. "We aren't wasting time staring at that worthless glass box any more. Life's too short."

"But, Mom, The Duke Boys!"

"You're going to think Duke Boys!" Whatever that meant.

We were not allowed in the house during daylight hours unless we had a bone sticking out, or needed to hide from someone with a loaded firearm. We rode horses, bikes, and go-carts; we chased cattle, rainbows, and my sister's friends; and we built forts to fight the commies, the aliens, or the sheriff.

In elementary school, I got good grades except for Needs Improvement conduct grades.

I filled a medicine bottle with water and food coloring and told my fellow second-graders it was "drugs." I drank it, acted weird, and collapsed with my eyes closed. The attention-seeking plan went awry when a boy tattled and the teacher thought I was dying. My parents weren't too happy, especially since I had tricked my mom into giving me the red concoction as a "science experiment."

My parents were upstanding citizens, and the most positive, honest, moral (but not moralizing) people I've ever known. My dad was thirty-one when he became a university dean. My mother was a computer programmer at NASA, then a full-time mom. She and my father worked on the NASA project to put the first man on the moon. Our home was a fine place to prepare my launch into this mean, happy world.

In middle school, I made bombs that blew trash out of dumpsters, and once burned up several acres of weeds; we skedaddled before the fire trucks showed up. I caught our garage on fire playing with firecrackers and gasoline. Whenever we were home alone, we drove the tractor at seventy miles an hour, preparing for our careers as Duke Boys.

God protects idiots, I guess.

We moved to a small college town in Mississippi. My Tennessee schools were all white; my new school was over half African American. They held segregated proms at the public high school.

My parents encouraged racial understanding. In ninth grade, I remarked to my father, "The black guys have sex at a young age."

My father's responded, "You can't judge based on your football buddies. Those guys are rough chargers. I doubt the behavior of the average black person is much different than the average white person." My parents grew up in the segregated south, but I never heard my parents speak poorly of any other race. They focused on building, rather than burning, bridges.

I played football through high school and benefited from the camaraderie. The team was over ninety percent African American, although no one used that word. I was white, they were black, but we were a team: the top ranked team in the state.

We were all buddies, but Fred and Steve were like brothers to me. Like Cannibal Cullison, both became a veteran of war, but he made it through.

Fred's father was a Methodist preacher and I attended their church when I stayed with them. Their church was the sister church to our white Methodist church.

When his father would bless the pork chops and collard greens, his mom would murmur, "Yes Lord. Umm-hmm. Thank you! Praise Jesus!" and Fred would look embarrassed and roll his eyes through his fingers.

Opening your eyes during the prayer was equal to cussing with a Bible open, but not as bad as making three Sunday school teachers quit in one year. But Saint Peter takes it easy on fifth graders. Hopefully.

I saw terribly racist things in that small town, in both directions, but there was more racial harmony than in most big cities, it seemed. Many blacks and whites in cities do not know each other, and this breeds division. Unfortunately, racial boundaries exist wherever there are significant numbers of minorities. Humans are tribal creatures.

In Portland, a bastion of liberal stereotypes, I heard nurses and doctors openly defame Gypsies. I remarked to another ER doctor,

"Everyone thinks the South is full of racism, but you'd never hear someone speaking publicly about black people the way people in Portland complain about Gypsies."

He responded without irony, "The Gypsies deserve it."

My junior year in high school, we decided to plan an integrated prom. Fred and I were co-chairmen of the prom planning committee. We raised money by charging admission to talent contests. Fred and I could breakdance and rap and we thought we were stars—nothing like doing the caterpillar in front of your entire school to impress the ladies.

Starkville, Mississippi, a University town, held its first integrated prom in 1987. It was a huge success.

My conduct still Needed Improvement in high school. I was happy, but rowdy. I snuck out of the house, crashed my car occasionally, and got in a few fistfights—more because I was bailing out drunk friends than because I was angry. In our little town, fist fighting was a form of sport, and a rite of passage.

Mostly we got into silly mischief. Fred and I visited the rival team's football field before the big game and left them an unkind message with a weed sprayer and diesel.

Another night, a group of us climbed into the University football stadium and shot bottle-rockets at the police station below. The police ran out and Fred scored a bottle-rocket explosion so close they scattered. We split up and hid in the enormous stadium. After an hour, a friend and I jumped the barb-wire-topped fence into the dark street that ringed the stadium.

A police car and an officer on foot were prowling nearby. The officer yelled, "Freeze!" and I responded, "Run!" and bolted across an open field, Duke Boys style. I saw the police car pull onto the grass and the officer sprint toward us. I ran as hard my legs would go for five minutes without looking back, then dove headlong into a bush.

As the joke goes about running fast enough to outrace your friend when a bear is chasing, I outran my friend. The police car drove between us and cut him off. He got cuffed and stuffed, but never ratted on us. His parents had to pick him up around 2 a.m.

Fred went into the Army and I went to Mississippi State, my dad's alma mater. I was a pre-med student but had serious doubts during undergrad. Doctors worked long hours, and I wanted a balanced life—I had a zillion and twelve interests. I thought about being a teacher, orthodontist, airplane pilot, or mortician.

After my junior year, I traveled to Mexico for a three-week Spanish class. I hung out with my Mexican tutor and his amigos instead of my classmates. I was the only gringo at Mexican nightclubs. I loved it.

I decided to stay the rest of the summer in Mexico. I went out with my new amigos and even had a summer fling with a senorita who spoke only Spanish.

A Mexican OB-Gyn let me deliver babies and sew up C-sections. When I first saw him pull a baby out of the womb during a C-section, I was filled with a miraculous sense of wonder. He cut through skin, tissue, and muscles. He exposed the uterus— buried like an avocado pit. He cut into the pit and pulled out a tiny, beautiful, squawking human. My experiences in Mexico cemented my desire to be a doctor.

My senior year, I fell for Missy. She was a laid back blonde with a smile like a sugar cookie. Missy was independent, outdoorsy, and thought outside the box. We saw the world the same way, laughed at each other's jokes, and got along almost perfectly. I found my soul mate.

Because I enjoyed my summer in Mexico so much, I decided to postpone med school to improve my Spanish and live outside the U.S. I found a job working as an Emergency Medical Technician in Paraguay and was granted a one-year deferment by my med school.

I graduated and moved to Paraguay, living with Paraguayan guys my age. While there, I traveled throughout South America.

I flew to the jungle to deliver medical care to a stone-age tribe. There was nothing—nothing—that they wouldn't do in plain view of their neighbors, the birds, the bees, or me!

"When you two are done with, um, that, come get your vaccinations."

Shortly after returning from South America, I asked Missy to marry me. I started med school in Birmingham.

I was drawn to emergency medicine for several reasons. I loved being Sherlock Holmes. What's causing the fever, the abdominal pain, or the tingly feeling? Those puzzles thrilled me in med school and thrill me today.

In the ER, the plaid fabric of humanity is represented. We see everyone: black, white, pediatric, geriatric, fitness freaks who push the limits, heroin freaks who push the needle, people with three homes, and people with three bags full of filthy clothes.

I liked the idea of limited hours; ER doctors work at a frenetic pace but fewer hours than most doctors.

The adrenaline is intoxicating: the feel of boiling electricity surging as we struggle to keep a sick patient alive. I've always been an adrenaline junkie, like most emergency doctors. In my younger days, I did embarrassingly moronic things in the search of an adrenaline buzz, such as breaking through ice to swim in the middle of a large lake, and jumping over one hundred feet from a waterfall.

The crackle of adrenaline returned when I was in medical school and we revived a man. He had been talking to us and then went unconscious—his heart quit beating and started fibrillating. We sprung into action. The resident handed me the defibrillation paddles, "Here, Brent, do it."

I pushed the paddles to the man's bare chest and said with false confidence, "Prepare to shock. Charge to two hundred joules. Everyone clear! Shock!" As his chest jolted and he inhaled a violent breath, I felt like I had wrapped the rubber around my arm with my teeth, popped my veins, and injected the smack that addicts live and die for.

▣　▣　▣

My final year of medical school, I decided on emergency medicine. I arranged a visiting rotation at Oregon Health Sciences University in Portland, Oregon. I had never been to Oregon, but I had taken multiple trips to western states: backpacking in Yellowstone, snow skiing in Colorado, mountain biking in Utah. I picked Portland because one of my classmates said it was the coolest outdoor city in the U.S., and the Emergency Medicine Residency had a good reputation.

Later that year, I arranged a two-month tropical medicine rotation at a hospital in Nigeria, and—as my last hurrah before residency—we also traveled to Europe and the Middle East. In Nigeria, I treated tropical diseases and visited rural tribes.

One muggy African evening, surrounded by mango trees and tropical birds, we received the news I was accepted at OHSU. Missy and I smiled and hugged. We held a party with Nigerian med students and danced until late.

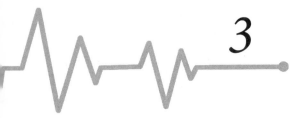

3

The first week in Oregon, I went on the Emergency Medicine Residents' retreat. We rafted the White Salmon River, near Portland. The scenery was stunning: clear water, rushing waterfalls, and glaciated mountains. I met my fellow interns: all unique, likable characters. Most had interests like skiing, mountain climbing, kayaking, and travel.

I sat on the raft next to Noah—my kind of guy. He was from Georgia and we talked about areas we had both visited. He had a flurry of loosely coiled blond hair, a contagious laugh, and a down-home, self-deprecating personality. He had gone to Vanderbilt undergrad and med school at Duke, but he seemed like a normal guy. His eyes danced like a man who had never been offended.

At the end of the day, we grilled and had a bonfire on the river's edge. The senior residents spoke about residency and imparted words of wisdom, but mostly we just hung out. Some folks got pretty loaded and the whole vibe was laid-back.

I was surprised at how similar everyone was: affable, relaxed, inquisitive, non-conformist, and fun loving. All had a myriad of interests and attacked life with both fists.

I have always been different than my friends; I was possessed by a curious spirit. Here, I had an odd sense that I had met my people—I found my tribe.

A few days later, I saw Noah at the hospital. He said, "You'll never believe what happened to me! After rafting the White Salmon, I decided to kayak it.

"I was by myself, which was a dumb maneuver. After about five minutes in the river, I knew I was in over my head. Way over my head! I was hanging on for dear life. There were giant drops and brutally technical rapids.

"I couldn't bail out because that section is surrounded by cliffs with no place to climb out. I was being pushed along much faster than I was comfortable. I dropped a ten-foot waterfall and entered a huge rapid with standing waves towering over me. I was scared.

"I got pinned against a boulder. I struggled to get off the rock, but so much water rushed over me, I couldn't budge.

"Suddenly, my kayak snapped in half! I got Maytagged in the swirling water: I was flopping all over the place. That water was freezing!

"I grabbed a rock in the middle of the river and climbed on. I couldn't swim to the shore because of the rushing rapid.

"After shivering for a few hours, I was worried. I wasn't sure if anyone would come. I was not up for spending the night on a rock. I was considering swimming when I heard voices and laughing in the distance. Five rafts appeared upriver. It was a church group. I climbed in and hugged everyone in the raft. Dude, I was singing hallelujah."

I laughed, "Welcome to the wild, wild west!"

I walked away, smiling.

I knew our choice to train in emergency medicine would be demanding, stressful, and grueling. I knew we were stepping onto a harsh proving ground—our constitutions would be measured. I understood all of that, but I did not anticipate the impact—like a concrete truck.

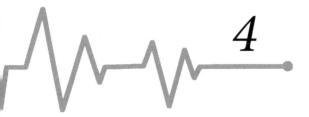

4

I was finding my stride. Incidents like Cannibal Cullison's outburst rattled me, but my recent shifts had been smoother. I made mistakes and holes remained in my basic knowledge, but I was learning and felt more competent with each passing shift. I became acquainted with most of the attending doctors and nurses, and that allowed me to ask them questions that were not covered in my textbooks.

The hierarchy of a teaching hospital has residents reporting to the attending physician. The attending emergency physician is in charge of patient care in the ER. Other doctors come to the ER to see patients and admit them. If a patient is to be admitted under a surgeon's care, the responsibility is transferred to the surgeon. Certain procedures are the domain of specialists. For example, an anesthesiologist is in charge of intubation of a surgical patient going to the operating room. At times, the lines of responsibility and turf are blurred, and this can lead to conflict, as I discovered this day.

Toward the end of a busy shift, I was finishing the treatment of a well-dressed, evenly mannered 30-year-old suffering from abdominal pain. I reviewed the abdominal X-ray, which showed, strangely, eleven one-inch spheres in his guts.

I went to his room to find out what he could have eaten. "Sir, you have several objects in your intestines."

He said, "Oh, that. Well. I have this thing I like to do." He chewed a fingernail, his expression flat.

I prompted him, "What do you like to do?"

He chuckled nervously. "Sometimes I cut off Barbie Doll heads. I shave the hair off and swallow them."

I held up the X-ray while he made this confession. Sure enough, I recognized the outline of Barbie faces. This was one cause of abdominal pain I did not learn in medical school.

"Maybe you should have told me this earlier?"

He waved his hand dismissively. "Never mind that. Did you figure out why I'm having pain?" Do you think it could be related to a curvy doll's heads clogging up your entrails? I briefly wondered what else he did for fun, but chased the uncomfortable thought from my mind.

I called the gastroenterology resident and explained the case. He said, "You gotta be kidding me. Barbie heads?"

I was tired and ready to go home when, thirty minutes later, my pager went off. "Level one trauma; arrival time, ten minutes." I groaned at the message. Nothing disrupts the flow of a shift like a critically ill patient arriving. Everything had to be put on hold. Missy would be eating dinner alone once again.

A level one alert indicated a severely injured patient. These patients are moving rapidly toward the eternal light, and a full medical team is summoned to keep them alive. A nurse told me the incoming patient was a middle-aged man who had been thrown through the windshield in a head-on collision. His wife and two children had been wearing seatbelts and were uninjured.

I was energized by the report. This sounded like a patient we could help. If a trauma patient can hang on until they arrive at the ER, they usually leave the hospital alive.

Still, that left me with ten minutes to do thirty minutes of work. Any patient that I could not discharge would have to wait until the trauma was finished, at least an hour delay.

I rushed to see one patient whose case was nearly resolved. I said, "Good news, your CAT scan did not show appendicitis. You have a viral infection involving your intestines called gastroenteritis." I wrote a nausea medicine prescription for her and readied her chart for discharge.

The next patient was a skittish woman who had been to the ER multiple times for minor complaints. I informed her that she had a cold and antibiotics would not help. She asked, "Could this be related to my neighbor's cat? I heard that cats give you a cold."

"No, cats won't give you a cold. Some people are allergic to cats, but this doesn't seem like an allergy."

She put an index finger in both ears. "I sometimes hear a whooshing noise in my ears. Whoosh. Whoosh. Could that be a brain tumor?"

This complaint came out of left field. "That's unlikely. You should discuss that with your primary doctor."

She was not to be dismissed so lightly, however. She wasn't leaving until she had received an adequate level of medical reassurance. "Is it unusual I have a metallic orangish taste when I burp?"

"It depends on what you have eaten."

Eaten any orange metal recently?

I couldn't waste any more time investigating vague medical complaints. A person who might be dying would arrive any minute. I fled from her room and flagged her chart for discharge.

The patient in room six would have to wait, I decided. I needed to tell him he had a boxer's fracture from punching a wall, but time had run out.

I hurried to the trauma bay, a brightly lit, large room able to hold twenty people. A single bed sat beneath a hanging surgical light, surrounded by medical equipment and monitors. The goal of trauma management is to discover injuries, stabilize them quickly, and move the patient to the operating room within thirty minutes of arrival.

I felt the pre-game jitters that reminded me of high school sports. Back then, while the coach gave the gravely serious pep talk, Fred and I would try to make each other laugh. The atmosphere in the ER was charged with a different type of electricity. A life, not a game, was at stake.

The attending trauma surgeon, Dr. Page, was the Chairman of Surgery at the university. He could be gruff, but he was well-liked, and had a great sense of humor. Sixty years old, he had served as a trauma surgeon in the Vietnam conflict.

By contrast, the attending emergency physician was Dr. Tom Vandeveer, a friendly but slightly insecure middle-aged man, small and mousy. He was my direct supervisor, but Dr. Page was really in charge, since the trauma patient would be admitted to the trauma surgery service.

The attending anesthesiologist was in her forties, a visiting professor from somewhere in Eastern Europe. She had a stiff countenance, like a KGB movie villainess. I had never met her before that night. Anesthesiologists usually stay in the background during trauma resuscitations in the ER. They are in charge of intubation, but a resident usually does the procedure.

My role was to intubate if needed, and then direct the treatment of the patient. I needed to call out orders and direct management. Of course, I was not really in charge, but I was learning to lead. I was nervous about being the leader in a room full of more experienced doctors.

Three or four nurses and techs, assorted med students, random nursing students, and observers poured into the room. At teaching hospitals, you can always count on looky-loos. Noah happened to be on trauma surgery rotation, and he strolled in as an observer. He flashed a silly gang hand gesture to me and smiled.

I heard the ambulance approaching the hospital. I quickly put on a plastic gown, eye protection and gloves. I took my assigned position near the top of the bed where I could intubate as well as direct the care. I heard the ambulance wail in the distance and felt my knees quiver.

The pulsation of the ambulance lights flashed through the glass doors of the ambulance bay, lighting the room with a red and yellow throbbing. I looked at the grave faces of those waiting with me, lit with unusual shadows of red, then yellow. The ambulance doors burst open and the breathless paramedics pushed the gurney holding the battered man. His expensive dark suit was splattered with blood and sprinkled with glass. His mouth was open and a gurgling gasp escaped, like a dying fish on dry land.

I made eye contact with the man, and in his desperation I glimpsed a soul teetering over the abyss. Then he lapsed into unconsciousness, hurtling downward. I did not want to be the last person he saw on this earth.

The paramedics and nurses transferred him from the ambulance stretcher. The team descended: nurses starting IVs, techs cutting clothes off, and doctors searching for life-threatening injuries.

My assessment was that the patient needed immediate intubation: placing a breathing tube into his trachea, or windpipe. All medical students are taught a mantra in emergency resuscitation, the ABCs: airway, breathing, and circulation, in that order. We first control the airway, then address breathing and circulation. If we jump to circulation before the airway is controlled by intubation, the person may stop breathing due to an injury or as part of the dying process. All critically ill patients need intubation, to support the patient by taking away the work of having to breathe. When a patient is near death, every bit of saved energy is important.

Breathing is assessed once the airway is controlled. A breathing problem might be caused by fluid in the lungs, or a collapsed lung.

Assessing circulation entails evaluating and improving blood pressure and ensuring that oxygenated blood reaches the body. Circulatory problems can stem from a malfunctioning heart, blood loss, or low blood pressure due to sepsis—overwhelming infection.

I had spent a month working with an anesthesiologist, intubating surgical patients in the operating room. I thought I had mastered the technique of intubation pretty well. Of course, intubating in the controlled environment of the OR is much different than the scrambling chaos of the ER. Trauma patients wear rigid cervical collars that make intubation difficult, and many have low oxygen levels so the intubation must be rushed. Facial injuries, blood, and vomit also can complicate ER intubation.

This was one of my first emergency intubations. I was outwardly calm, but I felt the pressure building inside.

That pressure skyrocketed when Dr. Page, the trauma surgeon, commanded, "Brent, intubate this patient."

All eyes turned to me. Luckily, I was used to stressful situations. I had spoken publicly in high school and college. I played sports, and I once dropped a pass that could have won the game, in front of practically everyone I knew. But those tests were trivial compared to the pressures of residency. I had to prove my mettle with a life hanging in the balance.

There is a saying in medicine: "Watch one, do one, teach one." This means you observe a procedure once, and the next time you do it. After one success, you become the teacher for the next person. Many procedures are rarely done, so there's no other choice. Nevertheless, the experience is unsettling.

On top of that, in the ER, these procedures are performed in front of a roomful of observers. I felt the pressure to be quick and flawless. I was expected to do so. Some doctors I had worked under were unnecessarily harsh and critical control freaks that would remove any resident who made the slightest error or even showed the slightest hesitation. They have a point. With certain procedures, like intubation, time is of the essence. If a patient is not breathing, the breathing tube needs to be placed in seconds, not minutes.

My adrenaline had to be kept in check. I needed to be fully focused, and I couldn't have shaky hands or a jittery voice. The balance point had to be exact—calm performance under pressure.

With that in mind, I moved into position. Suddenly, though, the anesthesiologist, standing at the head of the bed, said, "Wait, we need to assess him." She listened to the patient's lungs. She felt his pulse. She listened to his lungs again.

I thought this odd. As a resident, she had authority over me, but her instructions were contrary to conventional management of a critically ill trauma patient. Intubation has to be done first—the A of the management alphabet.

The patient needed a bedside ultrasound of his abdomen and an immediate CAT scan of his head to look for internal bleeding. If he had either, he would need to be rushed to the OR. He needed a chest X-ray to look for a chest injury. I wanted to regain control of the situation and bark out the orders for those procedures. I wanted to show that I could lead.

After a few minutes of her mumbling and futzing around, Dr. Page raised his eyebrows as if to say, what is taking you so long? I tilted my head toward the anesthesiologist.

He asked, "Why isn't this patient being intubated?"

She replied, "We must assess the patient first!"

He responded forcefully, "This patient needs to be intubated! Do it now!"

The pitch of her voice moved shrilly from alto to soprano. "I don't want to kill the patient!"

Her view made no sense; you cannot kill a patient by intubating him. You could kill this patient by delaying intubation. Intubation does have risks, but was clearly indicated in this patient.

Dr. Page said, "Brent, intubate this patient! Now!"

She said, "No!"

He was the chairman of surgery and I knew he was right. I had done a trauma surgery rotation and he was one of my favorite teachers. He told jokes and was rarely uptight. He was charismatic and warm, reminding me of a likable coach.

Yet the rules stated the anesthesiologist was in charge of intubation. Instead of being a team player, she was ruling her little corner of power with an iron fist. I didn't know how to react. As a new resident, I was used to being told what to do with a unanimous voice, not a cacophony of contradictory demands.

I turned to the ER attending physician to be the tiebreaker. He was my direct authority and I would do what he said. He was standing against the wall, apparently trying to become invisible. I said "Tom?"

Dr. Vandeveer was a nice man, but he struggled with indecisiveness. He could be painful to work with, since he frequently wanted a second opinion. As a resident, we would awkwardly have to call specialists, and fellow residents, for needless consultations.

He shrugged his shoulders and looked down at the floor.

Great, Tom. Just great.

I couldn't believe he would leave me hanging. He was either paralyzed by indecision, or he was trying to cover himself if this incident went wrong.

Dr. Page spat, "Forget it, I will do it myself!"

Unfortunately, this was like my saying I would build a spaceship. He was not trained in intubation and the procedure is not easy. To intubate, a doctor sedates and paralyzes the patient with medicines, unless they are near death and not moving. An intubating scope, a laryngoscope, is held in one hand to move the tongue out of way and to open the trachea. The scope is L shaped with a light to allow the doctor to see where to go. Once the tongue is displaced, the vocal cords are spotted. A plastic tube—held in the other hand—is slid into the trachea. The tube is attached to a hand-held bag or a mechanical ventilator to pump air into the lungs.

Obeying my superior, I handed him the scope and the tube, and he moved toward the head of the bed. The anesthesiologist remained rigidly in place.

He said, "Get out of my way!"

"You are going to kill the patient!" Then she hip checked him, basketball style.

He was knocked sideways one step, but he returned force with more force. He crashed into her with his hip, sending her stumbling about three steps. She hit a blood pressure machine and sent it rolling.

The room was stunned into silence. The only noise was the blood pressure machine's little metal wheels rolling. I had seen occasional conflict between doctors, but mostly of the grumbling, passive type. I had never seen open yelling, much less physical contact.

Once he was in position, he pried open the mouth and tried to intubate the patient. Yet it was obvious he didn't know how to proceed. He couldn't just stab down the patient's throat and hope he was lucky.

The absurdity of the situation was overwhelming. The Chairman of Surgery was flailing helplessly. I wanted to be somewhere else. Anywhere else.

Dr. Vandeveer kept his head lowered. One medical student looked like he was going to throw up or have explosive diarrhea.

I had no way to know the correct move politically. The fate of this critically ill patient rested on the decision of the shiny new resident, and I was surrounded by a room full of experienced doctors. Still, I knew that it was time for me to step up.

I finally managed to catch Tom's eye. Answering my unspoken question, he said, "Do it. He needs to be intubated."

That's all I needed. I told the nurse, "Give twenty milligrams of etomidate and one hundred milligrams of succinylcholine." The nurse gave the medicine, and Dr. Page handed me the tools.

The patient began to quiver as his muscles became paralyzed by the medicine. In thirty seconds, he was no longer breathing on his own. If he were not intubated, he would die. The room was dead silent.

I inhaled deeply, placed the laryngoscope in his mouth and pulled upward with all of the strength in my arm. His tongue moved and I spied the vocal cords. With my eyes glued to the cords I said, "Tube, please." I felt the tube touch the tip of my fingers and I grasped it. I spun it into position and slid it along the tongue toward the circular trachea. The tube sank in, and I connected it to an oxygen bag. We squeezed air into his lungs. Finally, I was able to exhale.

Seconds after the intubation, the anesthesiologist screeched at the attending surgeon, "What is your name, sir?"

He deadpanned, "I'm Dr. Page. Ask about me in the Department of Surgery. They might know who I am."

She stormed out, her face clouded with anger. I watched her go with a measure of bafflement. Did they have a different protocol in Eastern Europe?

Noah bugged his eyes and opened his mouth in an exaggerated expression of disbelief. I smiled. Having a witness to the absurd made me feel better. His ridiculous face immediately drained me of stress. I had performed the procedure successfully. The patient no longer had to breathe on his own.

I regained my footing and said, "We need a chest X-ray." The A of the alphabet had been managed and now we were moving on to B: breathing. The X-ray showed three fractured ribs on the right side and a collapsed lung. That meant he needed a chest tube, another skill I had recently acquired while on my trauma surgery rotation with Dr. Page. I said, "He has a pneumothorax. We need equipment for a chest tube." To the surgery resident, I said, "Please place a central line."

The surgery resident placed a large central line IV in the patient's femoral vein in his groin. A central line allows rapid infusion of fluid into a large vein. The patient probably had internal bleeding and the rapid infusion of blood would be tantamount to preserving circulation, the C of the alphabet.

It was my turn. I mentally walked through the procedure. I picked up a scalpel and placed it on the skin of his chest. I cut into uninjured skin, wounding the man in order to make an incision between the ribs. In response, air hissed from his chest like a punctured tire. I forced my finger into the thoracic cavity between the ribs and lung. Then I inserted the rigid plastic tube to remove air and blood from the space between the lung and the ribs, allowing the collapsed lung to expand. I stitched a large needle into his skin and tied it to the tube, snugging his skin around the tube. Surgery is like chemotherapy—they both wound to heal.

I said, "Please bring the ultrasound machine. I squirted ultrasound gel onto his skin and moved the probe around his abdomen. When I got to his spleen, I saw the dark swirling shadows of internal bleeding. I said, "He has a crushed spleen."

Dr. Page said, "Let's go. We need to get him to the OR." We rapidly packaged him for the operating room.

The anesthesiologist returned to the ER to take the patient to the OR, and this time around, her demeanor was different. She realized she had challenged the wrong person. I suspect she heard something like, "That's Dr. Page, the Chairman of Surgery! That guy wrote the protocols! You argued with him about intubation? You shoved him?"

She said meekly, "Dr. Page, we will have the patient ready for you in the OR." When you strike a king, you must kill him—or beg for mercy.

The patient was rushed to the operating room.

Noah said quietly to me, "Now, that was one wild rodeo. Way to hang on, cowboy." He shook his head in disbelief and hurried out.

I had my one last patient to discuss with Dr. Vandeveer. He and I both ignored the debacle. If we tried hard enough, maybe we could pretend it never happened.

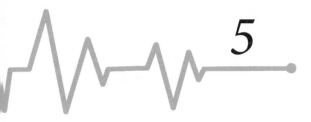

5

Since Missy worked as an elementary school teacher, when I had a day off during the week, I would usually do something outdoors with fellow residents. Noah and I were fast friends, just thinking about him made me laugh. His sense of humor was both wicked and silly; he good-naturedly skewered everything.

We were skiing on Mount Hood, near Portland. We both grew up skiing, but neither were quite Olympic material. We compensated for our lack of skill with enthusiasm and stupidity.

Riding up the chairlift, Noah asked, "What did you think about the debacle with Dr. Page and the anesthesiologist?"

"That was freaking hilarious, although I was irked at Tom Vandeveer for hanging me out to dry like that."

"That was pretty weak. I nearly burst out laughing when he started studying his shoes."

I said, "I can't believe they were shoving. General Hospital meets Ultimate Cage fighting."

Noah wiped snow from his goggles and changed the subject, "How do you like our class?"

"They're cool. Everyone gets along well. It's funny how similar we are. What do you think?"

He said, "I can't imagine a better group, with one exception— Franklin Trader is a gunner. He would plant his foot on your face to get a leg up."

"I've noticed that. I think he's insecure, so he boasts and brags."

"He's smart, eloquent, and dresses like Dapper Dan, so I'm not sure what he's insecure about. He seems malicious. We've all been around gossips and backbiters, but he seems intentional."

"If you and I have noticed it, so has everyone else. Gossips look petty and small. And here we are, being petty and small."

"True."

The chairlift arrived at the top. I said, "Let's check out the jump park."

He strapped on his snowboard and I pushed my ski poles. After cruising the park a few times, I was ready to show off my skills.

Noah positioned himself with his camera below a jump. I mustered my courage; unfortunately, I had more courage than skill. I sped toward the jump. The jump was a ramp with a thirty-foot tabletop and a down slope on the opposite side. To succeed, I needed to clear the tabletop and land on the down slope, where I would, theoretically, touch down softly like an airplane.

I knew I was traveling a bit fast, but he had a camera, so I had Kodak courage. I had to go big. The jump launched me into the air and my skis perpendicular to the ground. I slowly rotated backward, instead of forward.

At this point, I was not feeling real good about the whole endeavor.

I cleared the tabletop and the down slope and sailed through the air high above the flat slope, probably fifteen feet in the air. I hurtled downward, impacting flat on my back. I skidded and flipped like a crashing NASCAR, losing skis, hat, goggles, and poles in a yard sale of flying snow. My breath was knocked out. A long slow groan split my lips and carried through the snowy fir trees, like the wail of a banshee.

Noah rushed over. "Are you all right? Talk to me! Brent!" I couldn't answer. I made awkward grunting noises and grimaces. He thought I was paralyzed. After a few minutes, I was able to speak again, and I haltingly rose to my feet.

As he helped me gather ski gear, Noah grinned, "What's the last thing a redneck says before his death?"

"What?"

"Watch this, y'all!"

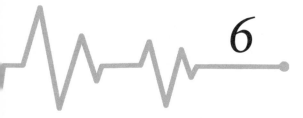

6

The first year of residency sped by. I spent almost all of my time in the hospital and saw Missy very little, but we both knew it was temporary. I learned more the first year of residency than any other year of my life.

During the second and third years of residency, we were given more autonomy. We staffed every patient with the attending, but they were much less involved with our patients. I felt more like a real doctor each day. The pressures changed, but as one thing became easier, another pressure was applied. No longer was intubation a big deal, but with increased autonomy, the risk of real patient mistakes grew. To injure, or kill, a patient was a constant fear.

Halfway through my second year, I arrived at work. I was pleased the attending that day was our residency director, Dr. Hans Maier. Dr. Maier had a strong resemblance to Sean Connery with a stout Swiss-German accent. He was well known in the emergency medicine world as a prolific author and expert. He was kind, funny, and friendly. He would play a big part in my life, even after residency.

Dr. Maier said, "Brent, this is your lucky day. You get to work with our star med student, Seth. Seth wants to train in emergency medicine. I believe he has a patient to discuss with you." Seth and I worked together seeing patients. He would discuss his patients with me, and I would discuss them with Dr. Maier before they were discharged. The shift was buzzing smoothly.

Seth presented a patient, "I saw a 45-year-old man who dislocated his shoulder. A neighbor's aggressive dog came into his yard and he was trying to escape when he slipped down. He reached up to grab the stair railing and his arm was pulled out of socket. Here are the X-rays."

I looked at the X-rays; the rounded ball of the joint had escaped from the hollowed socket—the egg had been yanked from the nest. I asked, "What are the three techniques to reduce a shoulder dislocation?"

He knew the answer; I was impressed, "You really know your stuff. I don't think I knew half what you know when I was a fourth-year student."

He tried to contain his smile, but failed.

"Have you done many shoulder reductions before?"

"I assisted with one."

We went in to meet the patient, a portly man with a white bushy beard—Santa Claus. I said, "We're going to put your shoulder back into place. We'll put you to sleep with medicines and reduce the dislocation. You'll wake up a few minutes later." We discussed in more detail and I asked, "Any questions?"

"No, I'll be glad to get this fixed."

We left the patient's room. I reviewed complications of reductions with Seth. I talked about sedation. "We have to be prepared if the patient is over sedated. There's a wide range of tolerance to sedative medicines. We'll use brevitol; it lasts about five minutes. Sometimes a patient will stop breathing, and we'll bag them until the medicine wears off. What other sedative agents would be appropriate? What tools do we need?"

After we had discussed the nuts and bolts, we went back into the patient's room. I held the patient's shoulder and Seth held the wrist. The nurse gave the sedative.

Seth manipulated his arm. I coached him, "Try rotating the arm outward."

I glanced at the patient. He had stopped breathing; the monitor showed that his oxygen level was normal. I said calmly, "Keep working on his arm. I'll bag him until the sedation wears off."

I moved to the head of the bed and placed a bag and mask over his mouth and nose. His bushy beard made it difficult to seal the mask on his face. I attempted to squeeze air into his mouth. The air leaked around the side of the mask instead of into his lungs.

I repositioned the mask; Seth was still pulling on his arm. I lost the cool, confident feeling of being the wise teacher. I swallowed my pride and said, "Stop pulling for a moment. I'm having trouble sealing the mask."

Seth looked up, concerned. I looked at the monitor; his oxygen level started to drop. Santa's lips changed as the liquid inside went from bright red blood—full of oxygen—to the purple color of stale blood.

I could not obtain a seal. My panic started to simmer. I told the nurse, "Get the airway cart. I may have to intubate him."

She ran from the room. I cursed myself for not being prepared. The airway cart should be sitting outside the room.

His entire face was the color of his lips: magenta. I was moving no air into his lungs. His oxygen level dropped like a stone. The alarms screamed. I thought, what's taking her so long? He would have a full-blown cardiac arrest if he went without oxygen much longer. I flailed. My panic boiled over.

I heard the nurse shout, "Where's the airway cart? We have a crashing patient!"

Several nurses and techs moved into the room to help. It was a small room; they crowded in and helplessly watched me attempt to force air into his mouth. The nurse rushed up with the airway cart.

She was in the doorway; the room was too crowded to enter. She frantically searched for the tools.

I said, "Pass me a laryngoscope." She fumbled and looked.

"Here it is!" She handed the scope to a tech; he passed it to me.

As I grabbed the scope, I noticed Dr. Maier. He was standing behind the nurse, frowning.

Jiminy Christmas, the whole world gets to witness me murder Saint Nicholas.

I opened his mouth and put the scope in. I could see his vocal cords but I had no tube to slide in. I looked up, "I need a tube!"

She said, "What size?"

I said, "Anything! An eight!"

She rifled through the cart; finally she snatched a tube, triumphantly. The people between us were not paying attention; some were starting a second IV, some were gawking.

I said, "Throw it."

She tossed it over the crowd. My left hand held the scope and I caught it in my right.

I slid the tube into his trachea—like a fat man squeezing down the chimney. I attached the bag and pumped air into his lungs. His normal color returned as his oxygen level rose.

I handed the bag to a nurse. I moved down to his arm. I pulled downward and felt the satisfying clunk of the shoulder relocating.

A few minutes later, he began to move as the sedation wore off. I returned to the head of the bed. He was breathing on his own.

I slowly pulled the tube out; he gagged a little. I stood behind his head as he woke up. I avoided looking at Dr. Maier but I could feel his gaze, hot on the side of my face. I finally looked at him when it was clear that the situation was under control. I was going to get a lump of coal in my stocking.

I said, "Sorry about that. I couldn't bag him due to his beard and the shape of his face; we had to intubate him."

He frowned, "You should've anticipated better."

"I know. I was careless."

He said, "No harm done. Lesson learned." He winked and smiled. He never mentioned it again.

The patient awoke from sedation; I said, "You were over sedated and stopped breathing for a few minutes. We put a breathing tube in, but the shoulder is back into place."

"Oh. O.K. Thanks for fixing my arm. I feel a lot better."

I walked outside the room with Seth. I said, "That's a great example of what not to do during a sedation."

He smiled, "Lesson learned."

⬕ ⬕ ⬕

I left the hospital. The soft Portland rain dampened my hair as I walked to my car. I was rattled. I almost killed a man with a shoulder dislocation. Even worse, it was the guy who knows if you've been bad or good, for goodness sake.

I was cocky and careless. I was not sure if I was ready to be out on my own in a year and a half.

I thought about a patient I had seen a few weeks earlier, a child with asthma. I gave her breathing treatments and told my attending she was ready to be discharged.

He returned after seeing the patient and said, "That girl needs to be admitted. She's working very hard to breathe. She'll be right back if we send her home."

I went to see her again. She was panting and had nasal flaring. I felt like I had been slapped in the face. Not that my attending was rude or insulting: he was right.

I reflected on both events with a sense of unease as I drove home in the inky night.

◻ ◻ ◻

The following day Franklin Trader was working in the ER. Franklin had a reputation of being a critical know-it-all, and was the only emergency medicine resident I found annoying. He dressed to impress, and flaunted his knowledge and intelligence. I had not had any negative interactions with him, but I kept him at arm's length. He seemed like he would twist your words to his advantage. I did not trust him.

I heard Franklin telling a med student, "Back at Yale, I did research on the pituitary function of diabetic mice."

She was enthralled with his research—a rich man's joke is always funny. I was entertained by the way he was able to insert Yale into almost every sentence he spoke.

When he saw me, he ran his hand across his slicked-back hair and smirked, "Brent, I heard you did a superb job on that shoulder dislocation the other day! I didn't know intubation was the treatment for shoulder dislocations! Way to go!" He flashed double thumbs up. "We should have all the med students work with you!"

The med student laughed obediently—until she saw that I wasn't smiling. She quickly erased her smile and looked ridiculous.

I ignored him, since I couldn't come up with anything witty or caustic to say.

Franklin was going to make my life difficult in cruel, unimaginable ways, even long after residency was done.

◻ ◻ ◻

A few weeks later I showed up for work and a nurse said, "Remember that patient?" My stomach flipped; those are the three most dreaded words for an ER doctor. Many of our decisions are based on odds and judgment. My biggest nightmare was to send home a patient who dies, or is permanently injured by something I missed.

"Which patient?"

"That Japanese guy you saw a couple of nights ago with a sore throat. Do you remember him?"

I swallowed hard. "Yeah. Did he come back?"

"He returned the next day and could barely breathe. He had epiglottitis and was admitted to the Intensive Care Unit."

Epiglottitis is an infection of the epiglottis, the flap that protects the airway during swallowing. The epiglottis can swell so much that the person cannot breathe, a strangulating death.

Epiglottitis is a true emergency. George Washington was killed by the horrible squeeze of epiglottitis. If the epiglottis swells enough, the patient will have to be intubated to protect the airway. Sometimes the patient's trachea has to be cut open so they can breathe, known as a tracheostomy. A patient with epiglottitis should be admitted, placed on IV antibiotics, and closely monitored as they can go south quickly.

I felt my face perspire. I mumbled, "Oh, wow. I feel terrible."

She said, "I wanted to tell you before you hear it from someone else. Everyone was talking about it yesterday."

I remembered the patient. He had complained bitterly of a sore throat. When I examined his throat, it looked normal. I had a vague thought that I should investigate further, but instead, I told him I thought he had a virus and should get better.

When I was in undergrad, my surgeon uncle advised, "Don't go into medicine if you can't live with yourself if you kill a patient. Not because you made an honest mistake, or because something was so well disguised that no one would have caught it, but because you were lazy.

"You knew the right thing to do, and you took a short cut or didn't want to get out of bed to check on the patient. Someone will likely die because of your laziness and if you can't live with yourself under those circumstances, don't go into medicine."

I was shocked at this advice, but he was wise. There are so many negative workups that sometimes we take shortcuts.

I had taken the lazy way and almost killed this man. I should have taken a fiber optic scope and threaded it down his nose and looked at his epiglottis. The hallmark of epiglottitis is a sore throat with a normal exam. If the tonsils and mouth are normal, the epiglottis could be causing the pain.

The only way to visualize the epiglottis is to use the scope, a time consuming procedure that is usually negative. The patient has to be very still during an uncomfortable, painful procedure. Patients hate having a tube inserted in their nose and often jerk involuntarily, making visualization of the epiglottis frustrating and difficult.

I asked the nurse, "Were you here when he came back?"

"No. I think he was admitted two days ago. Yesterday Franklin Trader was having a field day, laughing about it."

I grimaced, "What was he saying?" I didn't really want to know, but I couldn't help myself.

She unwisely said, "He said in the South they don't have new fangled equipment like fiber optic scopes since they don't have electricity. He was hamming it up, imitating your southern accent.

"He said you were trying to discharge him as quickly as possible since he was a foreigner. He said something like, 'We ain't got no use for foreigners in these parts! Yee-haw!'"

I smiled weakly.

⊡　⊡　⊡

I was angry and shamed. I felt like the chair had been pulled out from underneath me and everyone was laughing at my expense.

I read my initial dictation; I flushed with embarrassment at the simplicity and brevity of my explanation. It seemed so obvious in retrospect. The ER resident who saw him the second time was charitable in his dictation, but the admitting Intensive Care Unit resident's dictation excoriated me. He said, "He was initially seen in the ER and was told he had a virus, but inexplicably, no workup or investigation was done. The ER resident described a normal throat exam and gave no real explanation for the patient's severe sore throat."

The patient was not intubated but was still in the ICU due to breathing difficulty. He would be on IV antibiotics for at least one week.

I was unable to focus the rest of my shift. One patient said, "I already told you; I haven't had any vomiting." I wanted to leave the ER and not come back.

I felt the fury of the devil toward Franklin for his glee at my mistake. I could not confront him without seeming petty. He would act like I could not take a joke, and I would be pouring gasoline on the situation.

My blood boiled he would insinuate racism, especially since he was from an all-white, wealthy suburb. I remembered the last time I was this angry, in college. I was sitting in a common room watching television, taking a break from studying. Several students were drunk and one of them, a big mean country boy who lived on my floor and liked to fight, started berating the anchorwoman on the news. "Stupid n----r! Shut up, blue gum!"

My face flushed. I knew he was trying to jab me since I had black friends. I said, "Shut up, redneck."

His head snapped toward me and he said, "Who you calling redneck?"

I raised my eyebrows, "A redneck."

He stood and towered over me, "What're you gonna do, n----r lover?"

He was taller and heavier, but I sprang to my feet as angry as I had ever been. My teeth, my temper, and my fists were clenched as tight as a bear trap. I seethed, "The question is, what're you going to do, hillbilly hick?"

We stood nose to nose until a few guys pulled us apart. He left the room in a screechy bluster. "He's a n----r lover!"

I continued watching the news with a smile. The anchorwoman was beautiful.

◻ ◻ ◻

I left work and on the drive home, I tried to channel my parents, the most unflappable people I've known. I remembered sitting with my dad on our back porch. I was mad because of some childhood drama and he said, "Don't worry about it. Worry, regret, and anger are the biggest wastes of time and energy in life."

My parents almost never talked badly of others, and they would say, "If you don't have something nice to say, don't say anything."

My parents were masters of giving the precise word of wisdom. They weren't preachy and most lessons I learned from observation. They said not to worry with gossipers, schemers, and their ilk. If someone wants to waste their time thinking or talking about you, don't burn your time on their thoughts or words. If you care about what people think, you become their prisoner.

People think about you less than you think they do, and trying to make everyone happy is a fool's errand. Don't let people under your skin; there is only room for one person inside your skin.

You are in control of your happiness, since you are in control of your attitude.

They also said, he who makes you angry controls you.

Unfortunately, Franklin Trader was controlling me; I wanted to tattoo my fist with his dental imprint.

So much for the power of positive thinking.

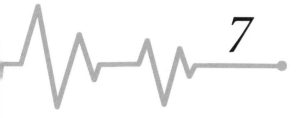

7

Two a.m. Weeks had passed since my near-disaster, but my thoughts were in disarray. I lay in bed, tired but wired. I had to be up for lectures at seven. I was exhausted but couldn't sleep. I was jealous of Missy flowing through dreams in her slumber. I closed my eyes, only to have them pop open again as the moon-soaked clouds filtered by my window.

One of the hazards of my profession is working evenings and nights. It's hard to be on the same schedule with Missy and other family and friends. I spend time awake with the strange creatures of the night: the owls, the bats, the truckers, the hookers, the raccoons, the cops, and the bad guys.

I stared at the ceiling, thinking. Being an emergency medicine resident was an exciting, but trying time. When I decided to go into emergency medicine, many people I respected tried to talk me out of it. My beloved uncle, the surgeon, advised I might get burned out. As I began my residency, I wondered if I had made the right choice. Should I have been a surgeon or something else?

Most of my friends from high school and college had real jobs, first houses, and a yard to mow. We lived in a cheap apartment and I spent my time being bossed around by cranky, sometimes geeky, senior residents with bed-head hair. The structure of residency was almost militaristic. I wasn't cut out for that.

Could I do better? Is there something that would fit me better? I could have been an opthamologist with respectable patients, a clean office, and normal hours. An internist chats with familiar patients who bring homemade jam. A surgeon removes a gallbladder and the patient is forever grateful.

ER hours are grueling. All residents work long shifts and have to be up during the night, but emergency medicine is a lifelong commitment to working night hours. The body never gets used to charging full tilt at 4 a.m. Late at night, the mind can play games. On a night shift, work that would be routine can be overwhelming. Fatigue clouds judgment and emotions. Thoughts entered my head I was not prepared to handle.

The politics of residency can be onerous. I'm sure there are people like Franklin Trader in every profession, but the mix of long, odd hours, limited social lives, and an all-encompassing work environment brought him closer, closer.

A few days earlier, Franklin and a few surgery residents were talking in the hall. He smirked at me. After I passed, he laughed loudly, as if I were the brunt of a hilarious joke. I wanted to throttle him.

Residency was temporary, but I was signing up for a life of this. Did I choose well?

There is a definite edginess to the patients we see. Drug addicts and the homeless have nowhere else to go. People up at 3 a.m. tend to be living on the brink, and they bring the brink with them. We see pus, blood, vomit, rot, death, demons, and hemorrhoids.

Emergency medicine is a humbling career. We see multiple sick patients every shift. Some are easy to diagnose; some are not. Some patients are treated incorrectly and they get sicker. Some patients are treated correctly and they get sicker.

Being an ER doctor is like escorting patients in wheelchairs across an icy pond—twenty a day. When the day is done, and none have fallen through, we can breathe a sigh of relief, at least until the next shift.

When one does crash through the ice, we leap into action. We yell. We run. We get ropes. We call for help. We struggle to keep the wheelchair on the surface; we wrestle to keep it from sinking below. We attempt to prevent more ice from breaking. We gather all the rescuers and we strain to pull them out. We try. We beg for luck, we pray for guidance.

We try hard.

But sometimes, despite our best efforts, they sink to the bottom— into a cold grave, into the icy hand of the Reaper.

The red eyes of the digital clock stared at me. Three a.m.

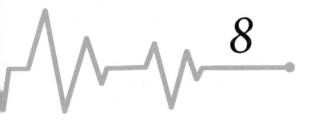

8

Occasionally, an interaction with a patient changes the way I conduct my practice. After I missed the patient with epiglottitis, I was more careful and ordered more tests. Sometimes a change can be temporary, an emotional, illogical response to a tragedy that is beyond my control. On the other hand, long-lasting changes can result from seasoning and maturing.

Rarely, a patient changes my outook, but Lillian was one of those rare few.

I met her when she was wheeled into the ER. She'd lost her balance, I was told, and fallen down steep concrete stairs. She couldn't stand afterward; her husband called the ambulance.

I walked in as the paramedics were loading her off the stretcher. "It looks like you took quite a tumble," I commented, trying to defuse any anxiety she was feeling. I shook hands with Lillian, and her eyes twinkled. Her friendly husband, Roger, reminded me of my grandfather, like he had worn a leather football helmet back in his younger days, Heisman Trophy style. He pumped my hand vigorously.

She said, "Doctor, I'm so mad at myself. I can't believe I did this. I feel so stupid!"

Roger said ruefully, "Oh, honey, it isn't your fault. I should've gotten those jars out of the basement. I feel awful."

They seemed like a sweet, loving older couple. "Where do you have pain?"

"The right side of my chest hurts when I breathe. I can't even think about taking a deep breath. I coughed a few minutes ago—Lord have mercy, I about passed out! My right arm really hurts."

Her description was helping me, but I needed to narrow down what types of injuries she had suffered. "Did you hit your head or lose consciousness?"

"No, but my pride took a hit. Guess pride isn't good for much anyway."

"Are you sure you tripped as opposed to becoming lightheaded or passing out?"

She was quite definite on that point. "Yes, my foot was tangled in my bathrobe and I missed the handrail. If I'd just been using the handrail!"

I said, "Let me look you over." I listened to her heart and lungs. I said, "Tell me if this hurts." I placed my hands on her body and applied light pressure to see where she might be injured. She winced when I touched her right chest and right upper arm. I ordered a chest and arm X-rays to look for fractures.

I went to see other patients while she went through these procedures. I couldn't imagine, based on what I'd seen, that her condition was serious. When I was alerted that the results had come back, I slipped into the small, dark X-ray viewing room. I snapped the X-rays up on the viewer box. Her arm looked fine, but her chest did not. I was surprised at the extent of damage to her chest cavity. I put the X-rays back in the folder.

I returned to Lillian's room. By this time her adult son and daughter had arrived. Judging by their hearty greetings, they were blessed with their parents' pleasant dispositions. I told her, "Your right arm looks fine. But you have four broken ribs on the right lower chest. You also have bleeding around your right lung. We need to put in a chest tube to drain the blood, and allow your lung to expand. You will need to be admitted to the surgery service for a few days."

They nodded solemnly. Stoic old-timers, they reminded me of pioneers who had traveled the Oregon Trail on wagons.

I asked the secretary to page the surgery resident, and a familiar voice answered:

"Hello, Ray Chang here."

I knew Ray; we worked together on one of my surgery rotations. Since it was a non-emergency procedure, I wanted to give him the choice of doing the procedure, or I would do it if he were busy.

"Ray, I have a 72-year-old woman who tumbled down the stairs. She has multiple right-sided rib fractures and a significant hemothorax. Do you want me to place the chest tube?"

"Actually, I'd like to teach my intern how to insert a chest tube. He hasn't done many."

That seemed fine to me. I had done plenty of them and I could move on to other patients. "O.K., she's stable. She's in room thirty-two."

◻ ◻ ◻

An hour later, I heard an overhead page, "Dr. Russell to room thirty-two, stat."

I was surprised. What could be the problem? I rushed to Lillian's room. Ray and the intern looked alarmed. Ray explained, "I'm afraid we put the chest tube into the liver. There's a massive flow of blood." I glanced down and saw the syrupy maroon fluid flowing rapidly through the clear plastic chest tube and bubbling up into the plastic box that evacuates air and blood. There was much more blood than the small amount that was around her lung. The blood was coming from somewhere else.

My nerves popped like a firecracker. This was a terrible mess, and sweet Lillian was about to be a lot sicker. The intern's face glistened with thin beads. I felt sorry for him, but much sorrier for Lillian.

I jumped in to help, all hands on deck. I ordered, "Start two large-bore IVs and run two liters of saline wide open. Send a blood count. What's her blood pressure?"

Roger placed his hand on Lillian's shoulder. "What happened?"

I replied, "I'm worried the chest tube was placed in her liver. The liver is located below the right lung. She may need an operation."

He nodded slowly, concerned.

I turned to a tech. "Please bring the portable ultrasound."

He quickly wheeled the machine in. I placed the ultrasound probe on her abdomen, and I saw the chest tube inserted partway into her liver and copious bleeding. The chest tube was sucking some of the blood out, but much was flowing freely around the tube, pouring around the intestines and pooling in her abdomen and pelvis, an expansive space that would hold gallons of blood. A belly full of blood would leave no blood for the rest of her body; she would die.

Ray was watching the ultrasound screen beside me. "We have to take her to the operating room. Page the OR!"

The nurse said, "Her blood pressure's plummeted—sixty systolic."

Lillian looked like she was falling asleep, decreased consciousness is an ominous sign of severe blood loss. I said, "We need O negative blood. Get two units here, stat!" My attending physician and several more nurses rushed in.

Lillian said weakly, "I don't want a blood transfusion."

I had heard this objection before. "Blood is very safe," I assured her. "The chance of getting AIDS from a transfusion is less than one in a million. The chance of hepatitis is one in 200,000."

"We're Jehovah's Witnesses," Roger said softly. "We're against receiving blood."

"Oh." His words felt like a sucker punch. My plan just got knocked out cold. I took a moment to refocus.

"Even if it's life or death?"

Anguished, Roger turned to Lillian. "What do you think, honey?"

"I'd rather die than disappoint my Heavenly Father." Her voice was weak but her resolve was firm. "I'm ready to spend an eternity in Heaven."

A nurse blurted out, "You'd die to follow those beliefs?"

Lillian replied, "Our Lord gave those instructions in his word, the Bible."

I had to intercede. I didn't want the conversation to deteriorate into a debate about theology. "OK. Let's use IV fluids and avoid blood. If it becomes absolutely necessary, we can discuss it again." I did not feel good about IV fluids since they do not carry oxygen and Lillian needed every possible advantage if she was going to survive this disaster, but we had no choice.

Roger nodded his head in vigorous agreement, but Lillian said, "There's no need for any more discussion. I don't want blood."

Roger looked deflated. "Does she need it, Doc?"

"We'll see what her blood count is. We need to control her bleeding in the operating room."

I walked to the nursing station slowly, sorting out my thoughts. I suspected Roger was not fully on board with the doctrine. That didn't totally surprise me. I'd heard about Jehovah's Witnesses who were willing to receive blood, but didn't want to be told until afterward. That way they are not culpable of the sin, but their lives can be saved.

On the other hand, I knew that people had been sued for giving blood against the will of the patient. One doctor had lost his house in a lawsuit.

Other cases came to mind, including one bizarre one. I'd read about a gunshot victim who was not given blood because he had a Jehovah's Witness blood refusal card in his wallet. After he died, the wallet turned out to be stolen. He was not a Jehovah's Witness at all. Maybe he incurred the wrath of God for stealing the wallet from a Witness.

One of our techs walked up. He had a thick beard, beer gut, and multiple tattoos. "I heard about the Jehovah's Witnesses," he said in a tone of voice that left no doubt about his opinion of them. "One time, I was in a grumpy mood. A car pulled in our drive and a middle-aged couple bopped out. They were carrying books and were gussied up in their Sunday-go-to-meeting clothes. I knew right away it was the Jehovah's. I was not in the mood at all.

"So I stripped off all my clothes. When they knocked on the door, I snatched it open, completely naked. I shouted, 'What?' with a snarl. They looked like they'd seen a ghost. They almost fell over. You wouldn't believe how fast they hustled to their car. They practically burned rubber out of there.

"I sat on my couch and laughed. I had tears on my face I was laughing so hard. My wife scolded me, burst out laughing, and scolded me again."

I smiled, but I was not really in a joking mood.

◨　◨　◨

Lillian was rushed to the operating room, and I returned to my shift in a state of complete discombobulation. I was on a roll with iatrogenesis— harm caused by medical mistakes.

While I was working through my rounds, another resident approached me. "I heard about the Jehovah's Witness. People are so idiotic! To refuse blood because of some old book?" He made a face like he couldn't believe such primitive people still existed. "Maybe

God will save her. Did they lay hands on her, or anoint her with oil? Speak in tongues? Call Salt Lake for advice?"

His cynicism made me uncomfortable for several reasons. First, Lillian and Roger were very nice people. Second, who is to say they are not right? Articles of faith are unknowable, and personal. Third, I was pretty sure he was mixing up his religions, showing his ignorance. Finally, she wouldn't need a blood transfusion at all if a rigid tube hadn't been spiked into her blood-soaked liver.

I said, "I feel terrible because it's our fault."

"I know," he said, waving his arms in disgust. "That makes this all the more infuriating. If she dies, that poor intern will have her blood on his hands. Religious people can be so stupid."

I replied cautiously, "They probably think non-religious people are misguided."

"Yeah, and they're wrong."

I thought, that's exactly what they would say about you. That is what conservatives say about liberals, Baptists say about Catholics, and Sunnis say about Shiites. So many are sure.

I was sure of one thing: I was worried sick about Lillian.

It is not often that I have patients whose beliefs directly affect their willingness to accept medical care. Anti-western medicine adherents rarely come to the hospital. Of course, there are cultural issues, such as the devout Muslim woman who does not want to be touched by a male. Usually these issues can be resolved with tact.

Religious views may conflict with science and medicine. Occasionally, they will adjust based on overwhelming evidence, as the Catholic Church did regarding the earth being flat. They decided that the "four corners of the earth" in the Bible was a metaphor and reconciled with science.

In this case, the evidence was clear that Lillian would benefit from blood, but she was worried about eternal consequences. Like the jihadist blowing himself up, the rewards are believed to be in the afterlife, and the sacrifice on earth deemed worth it.

Lillian had taken her entire life to become what she was, and to arrive at the beliefs she had. To think that I could convince her otherwise was unrealistic, maybe even arrogant. She had every right to choose her own treatment and control her own body.

However, it did not make it any easier to be her doctor.

◪　◪　◪

I called the operating room to check on Lillian's status. The OR nurse said, "They removed the chest tube and packed her liver. She continues to bleed, though. They worked a long time, but they're about to close up and put her in the Surgical ICU. Hopefully the bleeding will stop soon."

I hung up and felt a gnawing in my gut.

Not good.

A human cannot live without the liver. The organ is composed of spongy material saturated with blood and it acts as a blood filter. Stitching the liver is like trying to sew a sponge together while it sits under a running faucet.

They packed Lillian's liver with pads to assist with clotting, and to stop the free flow of blood spilling into the abdomen. There is about a twenty percent fatality rate for a simple liver laceration: for an elderly patient who refuses blood, the percentage was higher.

Much higher.

◪　◪　◪

At the end of my shift I went to the ICU to see how she was doing. I saw Ray, the surgery resident, sitting outside her room, illuminated in a fluorescent pale wash. Through the door, monitors beeped constantly.

"What's up?" I asked.

He ran all ten fingers through his hair and exhaled. "It ain't good. Her blood count continues to drop. Last hematocrit was nineteen."

"Nineteen?" Normal is forty and we usually transfuse elderly people when it drops below thirty. "I doubt she'll survive the low teens."

"Tell me about it." His head was down, shaking like he couldn't believe this had happened. "I feel like total stool. I was supervising the intern. We were using a trocar and we just rammed it right into the liver." I could tell he was replaying those awful moments. "I can't believe her liver was that high in her chest."

"I've never used a trocar. How does that work?"

"Not well, clearly." He sighed and used his hands to illustrate. "The tube can be inserted with more force because it's attached to a rigid spear-like trocar. Since she had so much blood in her chest, I thought forcing the tube would be an advantage." He dropped his head again. "I thought wrong."

Ray accompanied me as I looked in on Lillian. She was on a breathing machine with wires and tubes protruding unnaturally. The spunky grandmother had been slashed and torn. Like a broken egg with the yolk—the living liquid—drained, Lillian's delicate shell was receiving IV fluids—clear, watery, oxygen-lacking fluids. Those wouldn't be enough. She needed blood.

I asked Ray, "Have you discussed a blood transfusion again?"

"I talked with her husband after surgery. He was worried sick. But his reverend was there." Ray rolled his eyes. "The guy had blow-dried hair and a cheap polyester suit. Anyway, I told them she might not survive without blood.

"The husband said she didn't want blood and he didn't want to go against her wishes. He seemed conflicted." His voice gained some heat as he added, "The good reverend was probably dispatched to make sure that we don't give her any sinful blood. The poor lady is about to die and the reverend's here to enforce the rules."

I asked, discouraged, "What did the reverend say?"

"He didn't say anything, but I bet that's his role."

I wondered if possibly the reverend's role was to comfort the family and pray with them.

We all have to find someone else to blame.

▣　▣　▣

I went to the waiting room and found Roger and his family in a corner. The pastor was not around.

When Roger saw me, he exclaimed, "Dr. Russell. It's just terrible! They said she might die!" A wave of tears erupted and a sob escaped him. His daughter rubbed his back.

She said, "Do you know anything? How is she?"

I said, "Her situation is critical. Her bleeding hasn't stopped."

The son's eyes flashed with anger. "How could this have happened? How could you allow an intern to practice on Mother?"

I felt defensive, but I was not going to argue about a standard medical practice. "Dr. Chang has probably done more chest tubes in the past year than I've done in my entire life. He was supervising the procedure." I could hear how this sounded. Whatever was the right of it, Lillian was wronged. "I feel terrible this happened. I'm sorry."

The son said, "Sorry isn't good enough!"

Roger wiped away his tears and intervened. "Steve, these doctors are trying to do their best. Everyone makes mistakes. The good Lord's in control."

The son glowered like he wanted to punch someone.

Roger turned to me. "Is there anything else you can do?"

"I'm not directly involved in her care anymore," I sheepishly mumbled, "but the surgeons are doing everything they can do. Except a blood transfusion, of course."

Steve said, "Why don't we just give her blood, Dad? God'll forgive us."

The family went deathly still, like all the air had been sucked out of the room. It seemed Steve had crossed the Rubicon.

In the yawning silence I felt very awkward. I was a stranger to their beliefs, a newcomer on the scene. I was a witness to the sacred and felt out of place. Different than witnessing prayers, I was a participant in a conversation about a foundational belief that anchored this family's faith.

Finally, Roger exhaled loudly. "You know, Steve, if it was up to me, I would. I can't stand the thought of losing my darling wife of over fifty years. I can't imagine living without her. Your mother is such a good woman. Those grandchildren love their grandmother."

He fought back another wave of tears, and his voice warbled unsteadily as he continued. "But she doesn't want blood. If she were to recover and find out I told them to give her blood, she'd live out the rest of her time in agony. I can't do that. It'd be selfish."

His daughter nodded her agreement through overflowing eyes.

My eyes stung as well. "We'll hope for the best," I said, quietly. "I'm sorry. I'll check back later." I walked away with a clenched throat.

After hearing Roger's thoughts on his religion, I knew any further attempts at trying to persuade them would be wrong. If I were going to be mad at someone, it would have to be Ray, the intern, the founder of the religion, or myself. To blame Roger and Lillian for their convictions was too convenient.

Once again I contemplated my role in this tragedy. Should I have done more? Something different? Placing a chest tube is routine; Ray could do it blindfolded. Yet the only way for an intern to learn is to perform under supervision. I am sure that Ray showed him where to insert the tube, so the injury really wasn't the intern's fault. And we weren't wrong to allow the intern to place the chest tube; everyone has to do it for the first time once. Still, I second-guessed every step of what we'd done.

A former case loomed in my mind, concerning a teenage driver whom I had seen in the ER. She was fiddling with her cell phone when she sideswiped a bicyclist, killing him.

Should she be blamed for the death? Should the driver's ed teacher? The parents? The law that allows 16-year-old drivers?

What if she had been dialing her phone and had run off the road, but there was no cyclist at that spot, at that time?

Wasn't that morally the same?

This was a perfect example of what my uncle meant when he said not to go into medicine if you could not live with blood on your hands. If I had been in the room with the ultrasound machine, we would have seen the unusual position of the liver. If the surgeons had used the ultrasound machine, they would have seen its position. Placing a chest tube is almost always done without ultrasound guidance, but that simple extra step would have prevented this misery.

Errors in medicine are often multifactorial—many factors are involved: complicated cases, hurried doctors, and unclear lines of responsibility. Some errors are caused by a lack of knowledge— the doctor did not know that a sudden onset headache could be a leaking brain aneurysm. Much more often they are due to a lack of thoroughness—the doctor knew the headache could be a leaking aneurysm, but did not do a CAT scan because he deemed it unlikely. (On the other hand, unnecessary testing is a major factor for upward spiraling medical costs.) Some errors stem from inattention to detail—the wrong dose of medicine. Errors are more common in teaching hospitals in July, when the new residents arrive after medical school graduation. Errors are more common when the doctor is rushed or fatigued. I had been that way on plenty of occasions. Sometimes, when the OR is chaotic, surgical instruments are left in patients during emergency surgery, something that never happens during routine, controlled surgery.

▣　▣　▣

The next day, I went by the ICU before my shift to check on Lillian. The nurse said, "Her hematocrit continued to drop during the night. She bled to death and died peacefully."

She paused and smiled sadly, "I hope she is in heaven. Bless her soul."

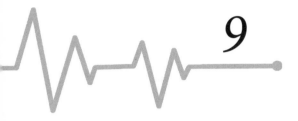

9

Noah and I ran down a windy dirt trail in Forest Park, the nation's largest urban park. We twisted through the forest of giant, moss-coated firs flanked with head-high ferns. I felt like we were little forest elves.

I told him about Lillian.

He said, "That's brutal. I'm sure the intern feels horrible."

"We all felt horrible."

"That story will make the rounds. That's one of the worst I've heard."

"Yeah, I wonder what Franklin will say."

"Who cares?"

"Did I tell you what he said after I missed the patient with epiglotitis?"

"Yes. You've told me more than once." He turned and peered at me. "Do you have Alzheimer's?"

"Probably. I may turn into one of those nursing home cranks that whacks anyone near. Maybe I could plant my cane across Franklin's nose."

"Knock out his sparkly teeth."

We descended a steep hill into a creek gully. At the bottom he said, "It's a shame to die for your religious views, but I suppose people have done that since the beginning of time."

"There were a lot of interesting social dynamics. Several people disparaged them for their religion, but I sympathized."

"You sympathized? Are you a weirdo?"

"They stood by their beliefs when it would've been tempting to adjust based on the circumstances."

"You're a freak. Of course, we each have our own view, but the Jehovah's Witnesses are odder than purple platypi."

"Is that plural for platypus?"

"No. It's plural for frog."

"Maybe they seem weird because we don't know any. Most people believe a version of what their parents taught them, and what their grandparents taught their parents. Unless you share the faith, or at least are familiar with it, another's belief system can seem odd. From an outsider's view, many of our beliefs, or lack of, seem strange."

"I don't have any strange beliefs...except that thing about being controlled by a tiny alien living in my right eyeball. But that's true."

I said, "I find other religions interesting, just like other cultures or traditions. I've been to Jewish and Muslim services. I went to an all black church several times in high school. We went to bizarre spiritual services in Nigeria. We even went to a voodoo market where they sold animals for sacrifice. Missy honestly wanted to buy all the kittens and turn them loose."

He turned around and looked at me like I was a purple platypus. He said, "The Adventures of Reverend Curious!"

I smiled, "My point is that different is not always bad. Different can be good."

"Maybe. But in the case of the Nigerian kitty-cats, and the Jehovah's, it wasn't that peachy."

"It's true that many beliefs are pathological and cause suffering. On the other hand, I suspect Lillian's family was closer than most. I don't think I'll forget them soon. I had a vaguely negative impression of Jehovah's Witnesses, but after my interaction with them, my prejudice was flipped on its head."

"Next time they come knocking, I'll send them your way. You'll make a fine Witness."

We crested an overlook. We sat on a rock to enjoy the dusk view. The Portland lights twinkled, the city sliced into halves by the Willamette River. To the north, we could see barges chugging the Columbia. Mount Hood, Mount Adams, and Mount Saint Helens— snowy sentinels—stood guard over the city.

I said, "I used to think of Muslims as angry terrorists. When I traveled to the Middle East in med school, I found them friendly and open. Their hospitality was unbelievable."

Noah agreed. "I know what you mean. Working in the ER is sort of like traveling the world. Mark Twain said it well, 'Travel is fatal to prejudice, bigotry, and narrow-mindedness.'"

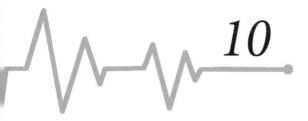

10

Noah and I got a kick out of trying to outdo each other in practically everything we did. There was no aggression or true competition, just sport. We saw each other often, discussing cases and telling funny or interesting stories. I was jealous when he mixed it up with Cranky the Clown, because he outdid any story I had so far.

◫　◫　◫

Noah was at work when he heard the paramedic radio. There was urgency in the paramedic's voice. The radio crackled, "We have a 34-year old involved in a roll-over motor vehicle accident. He lost control of his Corvette on I-5. His car looks like a crushed beer can, but he's not severely injured. He's banged up, but was walking and talking at the scene. I think he was wrecked before he crashed; he smells like a brewery and we found a baggie of white powder— looks like Ancient Incan Secret. His vital signs are almost normal; we'll be there in twenty minutes. Any questions?"

Noah said, "No, we'll see you on arrival."

"Hey, doc, one more thing."

"Yes?"

"Wait til you get a load of this clown." There was a shocking scream in the background, it sounded close to the paramedic.

The ambulance arrived with the patient. The paramedics rolled him into a room. He was strapped down with Velcro straps on a stiff backboard; he wore a protective plastic neck collar, and had a blood soaked bandage on his scalp. The lead paramedic met Noah in the hall.

He said, "This guy is a real piece of work. Get this: he's a professional wrestler. His costume is spread all over a half acre at the crash site. His name is Frank, also known as Crank the Clown. He just had a match in Seattle. My partner watches that crap; he says this guy is well known.

"He lost control and struck a tree. He was a seat-belted driver and the airbag deployed; he has a pretty large scalp laceration and his left elbow is injured. The car looks totaled."

Noah asked, "Does he have any medical problems?"

"He seems to have a healthy lifestyle! We found cigarettes, beer, whiskey, steroid pills, a bag of coke and some potato chips."

Noah was about to go off shift, so one of the other residents, Jordie, saw Crank. Noah dictated near Crank's room.

Jordie said, "It looks like you were in an accident."

Crank said, "No joke, Dick Tracy! You must be some kind of brilliant to figure that out! How old are you, about sixteen? Get me off of this board, boy genius!" He peered sideways; his head was restrained with adhesive tape and the stiff collar.

Jordie said, "I will as soon as possible. I know this is uncomfortable. Were you knocked unconscious?"

"How am I supposed to know if I was asleep? Sleeping people don't know they are asleep. Hello! Maybe I should have a different doctor. Are you a med student?"

Jordie asked a few more questions and performed a physical exam. He discovered that Crank was practically scalped; Jordie slid his entire hand underneath his scalp and felt his skull. When he pulled on a strand of his bottle-blond hair, his scalp came with it; he could see shards of glass underneath. The scalp was only attached on the right side of his head. He re-bandaged it to prevent bleeding; a scalp wound can cause very rapid—occasionally fatal—bleeding.

He ordered X-rays of his chest, arm, and the cervical vertebrae in his neck. He ordered a CAT scan of his brain.

Crank said, "Hurry it up; I feel like a roach in a spider's web!" He squirmed around, but was restrained by the Velcro straps.

"As soon as I get an X-ray of your neck, we can take you out of that collar and off of the backboard. I know you're uncomfortable, but it'd be unsafe for you to be out of the collar if you have a broken neck."

A few minutes later, Noah heard yelling from the X-ray suite. Crank was shouting at the hapless radiology tech, "You little punk! I ought to slap that smirk off your face. You were supposed to X-ray my left arm, not my right. Are you dyslexic? This is my right arm, and this is my left. Right and left. Get it? I got extra radiation! I'm suing somebody. I'm going to own this hospital!"

The tech mumbled something and wheeled Crank back to his room. Crank yelled and writhed; he was still strapped down. "Get me out of this! Now! I'm leaving!"

Jordie said, "Sir, if you'll calm down and cooperate, this will be over sooner. I'm sorry they X-rayed the wrong arm. We won't charge you for that. The radiation is minimal; you'd need ten thousand X-rays in your life to have significant radiation risk.

"You should stay in the collar until we've X-rayed your neck; a fractured vertebrae could leave you paralyzed. Your scalp needs to be sewn."

"I'm out of this cess pool! You med students can find somebody else to practice on!" He wriggled a hand free and began removing the Velcro straps that tethered him to the backboard. He pivoted into a seated position and herky-jerked onto his feet. He lurched forward wearing the stiff collar. He was enormous, probably six-feet, six-inches tall and three hundred pounds of twisted muscle.

He pulled the bandage off his scalp; blood streamed down his furious cheekbones, spilled over his hospital gown, and dripped onto the floor. He pulled his gown off; he wore tight underwear. He fumbled around with his cervical collar, but couldn't get it off. He spewed curses and incoherent blather; he spat a mouthful of blood onto the floor.

A nurse said, "I'll call security."

Crank had potentially life threatening injuries and was intoxicated— unable to make a competent decision.

Jordie tried to douse the inflamed situation. "Please calm down. We need to take care of your injuries. If you'll lie down, I'll suture your scalp immediately."

Crank kept trying to remove the collar. His bloody face looked like a horror movie; his crazed eyes glared from a crimson backdrop. He swung wildly trying to reach the back of his collar, appearing more frustrated by the moment. His scalp was flapping crazily on his head like a toupee—or a comb-over—falling on the wrong side of his head.

Noah told me it reminded him of a fire and brimstone pastor he had seen preach in Georgia. The pastor's comb-over would often flap on the wrong side of his head when he'd get worked up. The good reverend was constantly sweeping it back into place with his sweaty hand.

Reverend Brother Crank the Clown.

Hallelujah.

⊡   ⊡   ⊡

At that time, the University hospital was cursed with security personnel who had a mysterious grudge; many itched for conflict.

Some of them liked nothing more than to gang up on a mentally ill patient and tie him up like a barnyard animal. At most hospitals, the security personnel are professional and humane: hard-working people who do their jobs well. Not there, there was bad blood flowing.

My first year of residency, I witnessed an interaction between Noah and the security guards; my respect for Noah grew immensely. I heard yelling and rounded a corner to see the security guards hogtieing a combative patient. The unfortunate man had been permanently brain damaged in an auto accident years earlier. The security toughs had restrained his four extremities behind his back, with the patient lying facedown. This practice has been implicated in numerous deaths, known as positional asphyxia. When a person has that much weight on their chest, breathing is difficult. They can accumulate carbon dioxide in their body due to poor respirations, causing a vicious cycle leading to death.

Noah was twenty-eight and had been a doctor for about three months: a shiny new intern. They were older and had been working at the University for eons. Noah is generally a peacemaker and did not want to have an altercation, but we both knew hogtieing was dangerous. I was praying that our boss, the attending, or someone more senior would come stop the madness, but nobody came.

They were trying to subdue the man while he bleated like a lost sheep.

Noah said, "We shouldn't hogtie this patient; people have died from being restrained like that." I nodded my agreement.

The guards glared at Noah: exaggerated, teenaged glares with furrowed brows and down-turned lips.

One said, "He's a menace; his yelling is disturbing the entire department."

Another barked, "Who are you anyway?"

Noah did not give an inch. He stared at them, "I'm not joking. Get off of him. Now."

They hesitantly got up and untied their victim. They muttered and glared the entire time. They probably talked badly about Noah for weeks.

⊡　⊡　⊡

The Keystone Kop guards skittered toward Crank's room; sharks smelling blood, there was plenty. One guard with a resemblance to Boss Hogg said, "Sir, you need to go back to your room. Now!" The security guards had aggressive postures like street brawlers.

Apparently Crank's Worldwide Wrestling Federation instincts kicked in. He whispered, "Oh, yeah. I've got what you want."

He flexed his steroid-enhanced brawn. His clenched fists were near his waist with his elbows out; his veins popped. Blood was running onto his naked chest and shoulders. His jaw clenched, his teeth bared, and his eyes narrowed: sizing up his foes.

He looked like a bear on his hind legs; the stiff collar held his head forward. A wounded grizzly surrounded by yapping hunting dogs.

His eyes went from slits to bulging; spittle and blood flew out of his mouth as he bellowed, "Come on, pigs!" He rotated his head on the collar in an ursine manner.

Blood ran off his bare feet onto the floor, pooling. He took a step forward to leave.

They charged.

There were four of them and they averaged about five feet, six inches tall. The overeager first guard to Crank was clutched by his shoulders and tossed like Raggedy Andy. He landed on his back with a thud; the air escaped his lungs with an agonized hiss. He lay deflated and moaning.

Just as Crank released Raggedy, the others arrived simultaneously. Two went for his legs and the other grabbed his upper torso. He stood momentarily and then toppled.

They all collapsed onto a heap onto the ground. The security guys were slipping on the bloody floor as they attempted to subdue him.

Boss Hogg said, "What if he's got AIDS?"

Raggedy Andy got up and ran to join the party. He slipped as he hurried toward the pile and kneed one of his comrades in the back. They struck Crank with their fists on his head and back.

Fist smacking was not in the hospital security manual.

Crank freed one hand and swung his forearm across Raggedy's head, landing the blow to his ear. His pudgy face was pinned between an enormous arm and the bloody linoleum, tough day for the rag doll.

The security guards eventually got control of Crank; they subdued him on the ground and piled on top.

Gulliver and the Lilliputians.

One of them then pulled out a can of pepper spray and sprayed him in the face. He sprayed, and sprayed, and sprayed.

Crank began coughing, sputtering, and wheezing. Noah saw the security guards smirk at each other. He sprayed some more.

He cursed and struggled, "Get off me, you squealing piglets! I can't breathe! Get off me!"

After a minute or so, he lay very still. Very, very still.

Noah said, "Guys, get up. I don't think he's breathing."

One of them said, "He's faking!"

Noah said, "No, seriously, get up." They grudgingly got up.

Crank was purple and unconscious. He was not breathing.

Noah didn't know what to think; he was bewildered and shocked.

Why was he not breathing? Did Crank have a chest, neck, or head wound that had been underestimated?

At that point, he needed to be intubated. They would figure the rest of it out after that was done.

Jordie said, "Bring a stretcher and move him into a code room."

They lifted him onto a stretcher and moved him quickly into a stabilization room. He asked for intubation equipment.

He pried open Crank's mouth with the scope and looked inside.

Crank's airway was completely swollen shut. It was bluish and distorted beyond recognition. Jordie tried to pass the tube and could not. It was starting to look like the end of the road for Crank.

There is nothing that an emergency doctor dreads more than a patient who arrives in the ER alive and leaves dead—the celestial discharge. The inability to intubate a patient is the stuff of nightmares. The room was deathly quiet.

A nurse said, "His oxygen saturation is dropping!"

He pushed the tube against the swollen opening and was denied entry. He pushed harder, to no avail.

His oxygen levels had fallen past the point where cardiac arrest and brain damage occur. The cardiac monitor alarms were sounding.

He said, "Get an anesthesiologist! Where's Dr. Johnson?"

A nurse said, "Dr. Johnson is with a cardiac arrest patient! I'll page anesthesiology!"

Crank's heart rhythm became erratic, as often occurs before death. His oxygen level continued to drop. Jordie put a mask on his mouth to bag him; no air would move into his lungs. His airway had swollen shut.

"Get me a cricoid airway kit and a scalpel." Jordie prepared to cut into his neck to place an airway directly into his trachea.

This was going to be a last ditch effort; a surgical airway can be very difficult in a patient with a swollen throat.

He tried again. He saw distorted, swollen tissue. He suctioned saliva and blood. He pulled with all of his strength to get a better look. He saw a small hole; he wasn't sure if it was the esophagus or the trachea. An esophageal intubation would put air into the stomach instead of the lungs, a disaster in this situation.

He passed the tube into the hole. He connected the tube to the oxygen bag and shoved air in. The chest wall rose as the lungs filled with air.

A few nurses began cheering and clapping like it was a sporting event. Jordie smiled and wiped the sweat from his face. Crank's oxygen levels started to rise and his heart began to improve. He was connected to a ventilator. His pulse, blood pressure, and oxygen levels were all normal.

Jordie said, "O.K., let's do a CAT scan of his head, neck, chest and abdomen."

The CAT scan results were all normal. He was admitted to the ICU on the ventilator.

I saw Noah the following day and he told me the story. He was still unsure of what happened to Crank and why he almost crossed over to the netherworld.

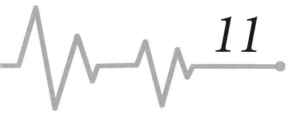

11

Waves rolled in from the Pacific and thundered against rocks, spraying foam and water. The evening sun lit the ocean on fire. I felt invigorated from an afternoon learning to surf in Cannon Beach, Oregon. The waiter brought us clam chowder, fried oysters, fish and chips. We sat outside, enjoying the salty air.

I asked Noah, "What rotation are you doing next?"

"The surgical ICU. What about you?"

"Emergency Medical Services."

"That rotation is cushy. You'll have plenty of time to read and goof off. You'll get a kick out of paramedic Ricky. That guy is a living legend; he always works with the residents. He'll keep you entertained. I've hung out with him since my EMS rotation."

"I met him once, when you were at the Lucky Lab Pub. I've heard a few of his stories. He seems like a clown."

Noah lifted his glass, "Speaking of clowns, I propose a toast to Crank the Clown and our humble and thoughtful security men."

Missy raised her glass and said, "I want to hear the whole story. Brent told me about it, but it seems too freaky to be true."

Noah told the tale.

Noah's girlfriend, Susie, asked, "What happened after he went to the ICU?"

Noah said, "They took him off the breathing machine the next day and he was fine. Everyone said he was nice, thankful, and apologetic. He probably had a reaction to the pepper spray, causing his throat to swell. I researched it a few days ago. Pepper spray is extracted from hot peppers. Normally it causes coughing, wheezing, tearing, and burning skin, but sometimes it causes swelling of the airway. There've been over seventy reported deaths in the U.S. from pepper spray since the early nineties."

I said, "You almost seem intelligent with that explanation."

Susie asked, "Why do they use it?"

Noah said, "They overdid it by spraying for so long, but he was out of control. Someone could've gotten hurt. He needed to be subdued."

I said, "The whole thing sounds like a tap dancer on crack. I saw Jordie a few days ago and he was still freaked. He said the vocal cords and epiglottis looked like a tomato. He didn't think there was any way he was going to intubate him. He was moments away from asking for a scalpel to stab a hole in his neck.

"I had that patient at the VA who died shortly after a big takedown, and it still bothers me. It would've been even worse if that guy died since he's so young. Did you do anything to help, or just stand around gawking?"

"No. I was like a war correspondent. I thought about jumping in when they had the battle royale, but decided against it when they started slip and sliding in the hepatitis soup. The good news is that Crank The Clown will live to wrestle again, and the security guys will live to annoy and terrorize the patient population again." He held up his glass for a second toast.

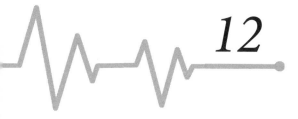

12

The next week I started my emergency medical services—the first rotation of my last year of residency. As an ER doctor we interact with paramedics daily. On the rotation, I rode the ambulance and answered the radio in response to paramedic questions.

Each profession has its stereotype. Doctors can be stereotyped: surgeons are aggressive, internists are cerebral, psychiatrists are quirky, orthopedists are jocks, emergency docs are nonconformist cowboys.

Nurses are strong, but compassionate. They bring warmth.

Paramedics are hard workers who meet the badness head on. They rush into stranger's homes, clamor into tangled cars, and yank gunshot victims off the seething streets with hostility peering from bleak corners. Paramedics, as you would guess, are most similar in personality to my profession.

Paramedic Ricky moved to Portland from a small town in Eastern Oregon. He was originally from rural Louisiana and reminded me of a few of my cousins. He was a salt of the earth type with a warm heart, feed-sack belly, and a friendly twinkle. He had broad shoulders like an aging athlete; he played football in junior college. We spent a significant amount of time waiting to be called and I got to know him well. We started meeting for a drink with Noah after work and continued the tradition after residency. As Noah promised, he kept me entertained with his stories.

He was on a roll.

He said, "One time we got a call about a boy having a seizure. There was a group home in the country for children with medical problems. Sort of like foster care, but all the kids had serious medical problems. The boy was sitting in the grass recovering from his seizure.

"After we'd been there about five minutes, several other children started dropping like flies, seizing. The children had run out and were watching us in the yard. The lights from the ambulance triggered seizures in all the other kids. It took us a while to figure out what was happening. One of the ladies who ran the home hollered at us to turn off the lights. They were all OK, thank God."

I said, "Yeah, flashing lights can trigger epileptic seizures. Many of the modern video games trigger the first seizure in epileptic children."

He said, "That sure was weird, seeing all those poor children seizing at once."

"I bet everyone was freaked. That must've been before there were good anti-seizure meds."

"Yeah, that was about twenty years ago. I got so many stories! Being a paramedic is nothing if it ain't interesting. I love my job! We get to help people and be entertained at the same time.

"Check this out, there were redneck neighbors who'd been drinking and watching a football game; these guys weren't smart enough to spit downwind. Their wives wanted them to trim the hedge between their two houses. At a commercial break, they hustled out.

"They picked up the gas powered push mower and held it above the hedge. As it was running, one of them dropped his end and got his hand caught. When he jerked his hand out, the other end fell and the other guy got his fingers caught.

"When we arrived, there were about four or five fingers laying around in the yard. We didn't know which ones went with whom, so we just bundled them up and took them to the hospital. I'm not sure if any were successfully re-attached."

I said, "Brutal. Alcohol and hedge trimming with a lawnmower isn't a good mix."

"When I was working in Louisiana, there was a funeral of some old guy in the boonies. It was country folk who kind of live out by themselves and don't have much contact with the outside world.

"They were all dressed up in their Sunday-go-to-church-meeting clothes. Those folks have funerals that can last half a day. Apparently the preacher was preaching and the choir singing. It was hotter than blue blazes.

"They didn't get the body properly embalmed and it got rigor mortis. The dead man in the coffin had a sudden movement of his arm or leg and thumped the coffin.

"Thud.

"Suddenly the preacher stopped preaching, the folks stopped saying amen, and the whole church got silent, staring at the body up front.

"The man had been dead for a few days.

"I bet you coulda' heard a sparrow flittering by.

"Apparently, his head jerked sideways so his face rotated toward the crowd. Can you imagine? The crowd erupted in pandemonium. 'The dead's alive! He's come back to life!' There was screaming and trampling.

"Pews got knocked over, there were several injuries. Someone called the police to let them know about the haunting. We arrived around the same time as the police.

"There were people running all over the place, completely panicked. A few of them had run so far into the woods, they didn't come back until the next day. The next day! When they got back they probably should've been checked into a mental institute.

"Can you imagine spending all night in the woods after being attacked by a ghost zombie dead guy with a rigor mortis smile? I wouldn't be surprised if them folks still ain't doing so good today.

"This one guy, who I think was probably not right to start with, was running around in circles around the church."

I said, "I read about that in med school. When a body gets rigor mortis, the head will often turn sideways as the muscles on one side of the neck contract. Sometimes a corpse will bend at the waist when the abdominal muscles contract."

"Sure enough. That's God's honest truth. That's what happened." He slapped his knee and laughed.

◫　◫　◫

I was an emergency medical technician in college. I took the course to help me decide about choosing medicine as a profession. I wanted real life experience. My first experiences as an EMT were part of my foundational choice to become an emergency doctor.

When I graduated from college, I decided to take a year off before going to med school. I went to Paraguay—in South America— to teach an EMT class and to learn Spanish. It was a powerful experience, living with Paraguayan guys my age in a tiny house with a dirt floor. My year in Paraguay was invaluable; I'm able to converse fluently with my Spanish-speaking patients.

While I was there, we went to a rural hospital to transport a patient who was not doing well. He was a middle-aged man who had an unusual infection no one was able to diagnose. He was barely conscious.

We drove back to our hospital. The other EMT, Carlos, was driving and I was in the back. We drove through Asuncion, the capital. Carlos liked to stop at green lights and run red lights. I'm not sure if he was perpetually confused, or if he liked the ability to break the rules.

Suddenly, wham! We were broadsided. I was knocked off my feet and onto the patient. He jolted off the gurney and both fell on the floorboard of the ambulance.

I was on my hands and knees, trying to stand. I heard Carlos cursing, "Mierda! A la madre!"

Crash!

We were jolted again as the ambulance was struck by another car; we had been knocked into the oncoming traffic. I flew across the ambulance, struck my head and shoulder, and fell on to the patient again.

Carlos let out an impressive stream of curse words.

The patient was bleeding profusely. His IV ripped out and squirted blood; he also had a facial laceration. I wasn't badly injured, just a few scrapes and bruises.

I helped him back on the bed and fixed his IV. The ambulance was functional and we limped back to the hospital. The patient's blood soaked my clothes and shoes.

A few weeks later, the patient was diagnosed with the first case of HIV in our hospital, and one of the first in the country.

I had to wait six months for my HIV test. The risk of HIV to a health care provider is not very high. The rate of transmission from a needle stick is only about one in one hundred. Hepatitis C is much more easily passed on to heath care providers than HIV. HIV positive blood on intact skin doesn't cause HIV.

I wondered if I could have gotten his blood on any of my scrapes. I wondered what would happen to Missy if I had HIV? Would she find someone else? How would it feel to be twenty-four and full of infection? To be filled with hoards of bacteria, having their way with my defenseless body?

To die?

How would I spend my dying year?

Life looked differently when viewed though that smudged lens.

I was tested at the county health department my first year of med school, in Birmingham, Alabama. A week later, the clinic called. "Mr. Russell, your HIV test is complete." I held my breath and waited for the answer.

"When can you come to the clinic to discuss your results?"

"Can you tell me the results?"

Long pause. "We can't discuss it on the phone. You need to come to the clinic."

I sank into a chair. It must be positive. "I'll be there in less than thirty minutes."

"O.K. Tell them at the front desk what you're here for."

My nerves rained sparks like a severed high voltage cable.

I mustered the energy to rise from the chair, and looked at myself in the mirror. My eyelid quivered.

I walked about a mile from my med school apartment to the clinic. I felt queasy; I tried to think of other things.

I sat in the waiting room for what seemed like an eternity: an inefficient urban health clinic. Destitutes and prostitutes loitered about. A few nurses sat behind the desk, painting their fingernails and gossiping. One man bragged about his third case of gonorrhea that month.

A nurse arrived, "Mr. Russell?" She raised her eyebrows like I was in trouble.

She took me to a patient room. She silently pointed at a chair; I obediently sat. She pulled my file and looked at it for about thirty seconds, the longest thirty seconds of my life. It was as if time moved slower the closer I got to finding out the answer. I was in a disrupted time vortex, a prisoner awaiting his death sentence, a blindfolded man bracing for the bullets, a head resting on the guillotine.

I wanted to scream, "Tell me the answer! No! Don't tell me the answer! Yes! No! Yes!"

She slowly chewed her gum. Chewed. Slowly. Slowly chewed. Blew a bubble. Popped a bubble. Paused. Chewed again. Glanced at her fingernails.

"Your HIV results are negative."

I stared with hostile intent, willing my eyes to burn, "Why did I have to come here for you to tell me?"

"Standard procedure. We like to provide counseling on HIV prevention for our patients. Did you know that using a condom during sex helps prevent HIV? Do you have sex with women, men, or both?"

▣ ▣ ▣

It was Sunday morning and we got a call from the ambulance dispatch, "Ambulance 41, to the Fundamentalist Latter Day Saints Church on Broadway. A middle-aged woman with a cardiac arrest."

Ricky said, "This should be interesting, that church spun off from the normal Mormon Church and they ain't normal. Hold on to your saddle horn, I could've been a NASCAR driver."

The ambulance pulled off, the sirens screaming and the lights disorienting. Many medics drive fast and loud, 'running hot.' They have the freedom to set the road on fire. The ambulance tore out of the parking lot like a prisoner at a jailbreak.

I saw a school age child weaving on a bike. I held my breath as we approached at an unholy speed; I white knuckled the armrests. The girl moved into the ditch on the side of the road and stared as we howled by. Her hair—and the pink tassels on her handlebars—swirled to life and almost came unhinged.

Ambulances are ten times more likely to be involved in fatal motor vehicle accidents than other drivers.

We pulled into the parking lot and clamored up the front stairs. A few serious men ushered us into the sanctuary. As we entered the holy place, I felt the golden Angel Mormoni blow his horn from the steeple—danger, intruders!

The women had their hair covered with bonnets and the men wore suits. I felt out of place, like a party-goer with a Goofy costume who arrives at a black tie affair, or the nudist who accidentally swims to the family beach.

The pastor was leading a group praying. Two church members were doing CPR on a woman lying between pews. The woman's face had a bluish hue; she was not breathing. We dropped to our knees beside her.

Ricky asked, "What happened?"

Someone said, "She collapsed during the service. She hit the floor with a thud. She wasn't breathing and Brother Joe started CPR."

I felt her neck. "She has a faint pulse."

Ricky prepared to intubate. He untied the bonnet below her chin, opened her mouth, and peered inside. I saw his eyes widen. He reached in and pulled out a flimsy plastic square.

The parishioners appeared confused; so was I. Ricky seemed to know.

Paramedics, like all emergency workers, see the dark underbelly of society—the destructive pathology that undercuts human existence.

He said, "It's a fentanyl patch. Hand me that." I passed the medicine bag.

A few seconds after he injected the medicine, she started to breathe. She was completely awake and lucid before a minute had passed.

The pastor said, "Praise God! Thank you, Lord!"

The plastic was a narcotic patch that released fentanyl into the body slowly over seventy-two hours, often used for chronic pain or cancer patients. The patient chewed it to release the medicine immediately.

Ricky gave her Narcan, which reverses narcotic overdoses.

She was getting high in church, and she almost crashed the Pearly Gates while stoned. Not sure what St. Peter and the gang would say about that.

We loaded her onto the gurney to transport her to a hospital. She needed to be monitored for a few hours to ensure she didn't become deeply sedated again.

Ricky whispered, "I guess their rule book doesn't let them drink, dance, or smoke, but chewing on a narcotic patch like a cow chews its cud is okie-dokie."

◘　◘　◘

Ricky was a paramedic, which takes significantly more training than an EMT. An EMT takes about forty hours of training, versus a two-year paramedic degree. Ricky's small town slang disguised a smart man; I suspect he would've been successful in any profession.

After our Mormon Temple invasion, Ricky told me about a patient who had a seizure at a nice restaurant.

He arrived and was met at the restaurant entrance by EMT firefighters. Firemen often arrive and perform first aid until paramedics arrive. One of the firemen said, "There are several guys taking care of the patient. He's a drunk who had a seizure."

There are many causes of seizures, but all involve abnormal electrical activity in the brain. The brain is a computer with electrical signals zipping around.

Senator Ted Kennedy had seizures because he had a brain tumor—like wiring random extra pieces on a computer; misfiring is inevitable.

Permanently faulty wiring in the brain causes epilepsy. Seizures can be caused by trauma, strokes, medicines, street drugs—anything that causes temporary or permanent brain damage.

A heavy drinker will be prone to seizures if they go without alcohol for too long. An alcoholic's brain becomes conditioned to alcohol. The withdrawal of alcohol, a sedative, causes an abnormally high level of electrical activity in the brain. The increased wattage causes seizures, known as alcohol withdrawal seizures.

Ricky rolled the gurney into the restaurant: hardwood flooring, dim lighting, and constipated waiters. The patient was standing, slumped forward with his arms over the shoulders of two firemen. The family was standing by. The wait staff looked anxious in their dark jackets and cocktail dresses; seizures and firemen didn't exactly mix with crème brulee and whispers.

One of the firemen said, "This is Al. He had a seizure and we're waiting for him to wake up."

After a seizure, there is a post seizure recovery period, a deep, deep sleep, like a coma. What goes up must come down; the longer and more violent the seizure, the more prolonged and deeper the sleeping phase.

There are multiple types of seizures. The most common is a tonic-clonic, or grand mal, seizure. A tonic-clonic seizure—the perfect electrical storm of the brain—involves rhythmic rapid movements of the entire body. The brain is exploding, a fire spreading through a shed filled with gasoline and spray paint cans.

A partial seizure involves only one part of the body—one leg shakes like Elvis. There is usually no loss of consciousness and no sleeping phase; only part of the brain is affected—a contained fire.

The upstairs bedroom is in flames, but the rest of the household is watching television and folding laundry.

With a petit mal seizure, the patient stares blankly with momentary loss of consciousness but no abnormal movements. A petit mal is often unnoticed. Sometimes a patient will be talking, pause and stare off, and then resume mid-sentence—a car backfires and then cruises on down the block.

Pseudoseizures are non-epileptic or psychiatric seizures. The patient will buck their torso and wildly flail their arms and legs. Most people with pseudoseizures are not faking it, but the pseudoseizures are caused by psychiatric distress. It is usually easy to distinguish seizures from pseudoseizures by the movement—a patient with a pseudoseizure flops around like a fish in the bottom of a boat, whereas a grand mal seizure causes much faster and smaller movements—a stick caught in the boat propeller.

The EMT continued, "According to his family, he's a pretty heavy drinker."

Ricky noticed there were multiple alcoholic drinks on his table. He found that curious since alcoholic seizures are caused by alcohol withdrawal—maybe the drinks were not the patient's?

Ricky asked, "What happened?"

The fireman said, "About fifteen minutes ago, Al went to the bathroom. Someone heard him fall in the restroom. They checked on him and he was seizing. When we arrived he was lying in the floor unconscious.

"He's out of it. We're just holding him until he wakes up a little bit. It didn't seem right to leave him lying on the ground." The EMT shifted and Al's head rolled loosely, like dead weight.

Ricky asked, "Does he have a history of seizures? Has he recently quit drinking?"

"No, they said this was his first seizure. I'm pretty sure that he quit drinking," he paused and grinned widely, "about fifteen minutes ago."

Ricky felt uneasy; it wasn't making sense. He walked over and put his stethoscope on Al's chest.

He didn't hear anything. He felt for a carotid pulse on his neck. Nothing.

He said, "Lay him down. He's in cardiac arrest."

The EMTs looked confused and lowered the patient to the floor.

Ricky said, "Start chest compressions. We need to intubate him."

Ricky was perplexed. What happened? It's almost unheard of to have a cardiac arrest from a seizure. Maybe he had a heart attack, went into cardiac arrest, and had a seizure?

The last scenario seemed unlikely; seizures can happen as the brain loses oxygen, but a seizure is brief in a cardiac arrest scenario, usually just seconds.

He grabbed a laryngoscope. He opened the patient's mouth and peered inside. There was something blocking his view. He pulled harder.

There was a piece of filet mignon wedged in Al's throat. Ricky pulled it out with forceps.

There were gasps and murmurs from the onlookers.

The reality hit Ricky like a bullet to the cranium—Al was drinking, and attempted to swallow a poorly chewed piece of meat. His family had not realized he was choking. He stood up, went to the rest room, and collapsed on the floor. The lack of oxygen caused him to seize.

The lack of oxygen caused him to die.

Ricky intubated Al and continued CPR. They moved him onto the gurney and into the ambulance. When he was hooked to a cardiac monitor, his heart rhythm was flat-lined, indicating that he had been dead for a while. They performed CPR and gave resuscitation drugs, but it was futile. He had been dead too long.

They declared him dead in the ambulance.

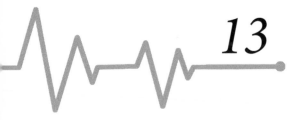

My EMS rotation was finished. I was impressed with Ricky and most of the paramedics. We worked a few auto accidents where the people were destroyed: mangled and ripped to shreds, faces and body parts missing. I had nightmares while Ricky took it in stride; he was used to it. In the ER, our chaos is more controlled, and mangled bodies go the morgue, not the ER.

I was at our weekly resident conference: three hours of lectures on a variety of topics and an hour-long Morbidity and Mortality conference: interesting cases, mismanaged cases, or cases with unfortunate outcomes. We had already heard two lectures: eye injuries and the management of congestive heart failure.

I was asked to present the case of Mr. Cullison in the M and M conference. It had been over a year earlier, but went well with the lecture on congestive heart failure. His death needed to be reviewed and evaluated, especially since it happened after an altercation with security.

The conferences can be brutal: an inquisition. The presenter is often grilled with complicated questions. If I didn't know the answer, I would look silly and unprepared. There were over one hundred people in attendance: medical students, nurses, residents, and attending physicians. I was nervous, but I tried to concentrate on the lectures.

The last lecture was on medical malpractice lawsuits. There was much interest in the dreaded lawsuit. Dr. Maier, our residency director, was an engaging speaker and his lectures were always favorites: full of experience, sprinkled with anecdotes.

Dr. Maier was a primary editor of a major Emergency Medicine textbook. He was cheerful and upbeat, and the residents felt he had our best interest in mind. His opinion was key to getting a good job; he knew doctors all over the West, and had a highly valued opinion.

Dr. Maier began, "To avoid being sued, you should be careful, and maintain good communication with your patients. Judgment errors are inevitable. We all make our best decisions based on the information we have, and our imperfect calculations of the odds. When you see thousands of patients per year, you will be wrong occasionally.

"If there's a bad outcome, the doctors who are liked by their patients are much less likely to be sued. Nevertheless, most emergency physicians get sued once or twice in their career.

"In a lawsuit, the plaintiff's lawyer will try to make you look as sloppy and uncaring as possible, in order to sway the jury. You can protect yourself with good documentation. Explain your decision making process in your dictations. For example, you see a patient with a very small chance of appendicitis and you decide not to obtain a CAT scan. You'll be much better off if you have a sentence in your dictation that says, 'I decided against a CAT scan due to the very low chance of this being appendicitis due to the absence of fever, nausea, and vomiting, as well as the potential danger of kidney damage from CT contrast dye.' Good documentation can keep a case out of a courtroom.

"The plaintiff's lawyer needs a doctor who'll testify you committed malpractice. It's not difficult for them to find a doctor who'll do this; there are hired guns traveling the country to testify against fellow physicians. For some of these people, it's a full time job. Of course, these mercenaries have limited creditability with the jury; the defense will ask how many trials they've testified in, and how often they testified for the defense.

"If a doctor truly committed malpractice, it won't be hard to find doctors willing to say so. There's a place for physicians to help patients obtain justice and weed out problem doctors. There is a need for competent physicians to testify, or else our profession loses credibility. But I recommend against testifying against fellow physicians in your own town.

"If you testify in your town, you might be considered a money hungry cannibal. I'm not saying that's a fair attitude, but the community of physicians is like a team; don't attack your own team in public. There are fifty states in our fair union, no need to testify against people in the community where you practice. We have a saying in Switzerland, Sheiß nicht in deinem Bett. In English, do not empty your bowels in your own bed."

The lecture made me grumpy; my stomach churned thinking of a patient being injured because of my mistake. I cringed to think about a patient being so angry they would sue. I detest conflict and this sounded like conflict on steroids. I hoped that I would never be sued, but I knew it was naïve. Might as well hope to never grow old, or for world peace.

Our M and M conference started after a short break. I discussed the case of Cannibal Cullison and his unexpected death. After my fifteen-minute presentation, the floor was opened to questions.

One of the faculty asked, "What data is there on bumex versus lasix in a patient with end stage congestive heart failure?"

I had studied in preparation for my talk and had a satisfactory answer.

Another said, "You didn't tell us what the patient's jugular veins looked like. Don't you think that is pertinent information for the evaluation of CHF?"

I responded, "Sorry, I failed to mention that. His jugular veins were engorged to the level of his jaw."

Another doctor asked, "Why would you use dopamine in this patient?"

After about fifteen minutes of being grilled, I thought I had survived satisfactorily. From the sea of faces, one more hand was raised.

Franklin Trader.

As soon as I saw his hand, a flame surged, casting my satisfaction in smoky shadows. He had an earnest, concerned look on his smarmy pale face. Usually fellow residents tossed out softball questions or made affirming comments. Franklin was known to go for the throat.

He said, "It would seem to me that an emergency medicine resident should be able to anticipate a sudden death event. I know you were an intern when this happened, but we learned those types of things in med school.

"Plain old common sense would say it's dangerous to have a critically ill patient involved in a violent altercation with security. Would you let the security goons attack your ailing father?

"Also, why didn't you get a second EKG after the out-of-control fiasco?"

There were snickers and gasps.

I flashed angry, then willed the fury into submission. I stood quietly and stared at him. The ruckus quickly died; it was apparent I was annoyed.

I toyed with the idea of not answering him, but I thought that might make me look like a thin-skinned hot head or a grudge holder. Better to play the nice guy and let the audience judge his intent.

I said, "Of course, hindsight is twenty-twenty, but you have a good point. I probably should've asked for a different security guard after the first squabble. That might've eased the tension.

"He wasn't complaining of chest pain, so I never considered a second EKG."

After the conference, Noah walked up, "Franklin is such a simpering pile of stool. Doesn't he realize he looks like a cutthroat?"

I replied, "I don't want to let that guy get to me. A few more months and I'll never have to see him again. He's smart as a whip, but his ambition is getting the best of him, or the best of me.

"I had an overwhelming urge to fling my clipboard at him like a Frisbee."

Noah laughed, "That would've been the greatest moment of my life: you fling it and smash his nose. He falls from his seat and you ask, 'any more questions from the audience?'"

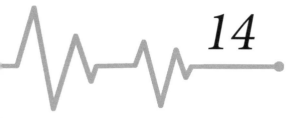

14

For the final six months of my residency, I had nothing left but ER rotations. During my residency, I rotated on general surgery, trauma surgery, internal medicine, anesthesia, emergency medical services, toxicology, obstetrics, as well as almost half a year working in intensive care units: pediatric, surgical, cardiac, and general medical. I was on the home stretch, but I still had a long way to go.

My shift was halfway through. I had a patient with possible appendicitis. He was thirty, with one day of abdominal pain and vomiting. He hurt diffusely throughout his abdomen, but was most tender in his right lower abdomen, the location of his appendix.

He had normal lab and urine tests, except for a slight elevation of his white blood cell count. Many problems, including appendicitis, will cause an elevation of the white blood cell count. The CAT scan was inconclusive; the appendix was not visualized. I discussed the case with my attending and decided to consult surgery. The options were to discharge him with close follow up, admit him for serial exams and observation, or to perform surgery.

Missing appendicitis, or waiting too long to do surgery, is to be avoided at all costs. The appendix, about the size of a finger, slowly swells like a little balloon. When it bursts, liquid stool and foul fecal bacteria splatter into the nooks and crannies of the sterile abdominal cavity causing pus, adhesions, inflammation, abscess formation, and misery.

Fifty years ago a ruptured appendix was a death sentence. Surgery on a ruptured appendix is complicated. The abdominal incision cannot be closed; the patient will have a gaping wound for weeks. Long-term pain and scarring are inevitable. The patient will heal slowly, over months.

I paged the surgery resident. Overhead page, "Line three, Dr. Smith from surgery."

I answered the phone, "Hello, this is Brent Russell, one of the emergency residents. Are you the surgery resident?"

Long pause. No answer.

I said, "Hello?"

"Yeah, what do you want?"

"Are you the surgery resident?"

Prolonged delay. Like a ruler on a desk, he snapped, "I said yes. What do you want?"

I was a little rattled, "I have a 30-year-old male with possible appendicitis." I told him the details.

"I will say it again, what do you want?"

"We want a surgical consult regarding discharge, admission for observation, or surgery."

Click.

"Hello? Hello?" I looked at the cordless phone to see if the power was on. I wasn't sure if I should call him back.

Twenty minutes later, I saw him leave the patient's room. He walked out, sat down, and began writing his note.

I walked over, "Are you the surgery resident? Thanks for coming to see him."

Without looking up, he sighed and waved the back of his hand, dismissively, "Send him home. He doesn't have appendicitis."

"Do you want him to follow up in surgery clinic tomorrow?"

"Whatever. He doesn't have appendicitis."

I felt my inner redneck awake. "Why don't you think he has appendicitis?"

"You people in the ER just kill me. Can't you make a decision? It's obvious he has an intestinal virus. This is a waste of my time."

Surgeons, not always right, but never in doubt.

I said, "You don't know for certain he doesn't have appendicitis. The studies show he has a thirty-five percent chance of having appendicitis, based on his physical exam and lab findings."

I invented that statistic, but it was probably true, more or less.

He smirked, "If you know so much, what did you call me for? The ABCs of emergency medicine: airway, breathing, consult."

I felt hot blood under my cheeks. I thought, Congratulations. You have your little inch of power after being a geek your whole life.

Stand up.

Let's go. Toe to toe. Me and you.

You want to tangle? Lock horns?

Get up. Let's settle this the old way.

What do you think about that, smirky-pants?

It would be hard to explain a doctor brawl to my residency director.

Maybe I should just grab an ear and twist.

Or fake a trip and fall on him. Clumsily clamor all over him as I'm trying to get up. "Oh, I'm so sorry. How embarrassing!" Push on his face as I get up.

He continued to write while I glared at his hair. I gave up and walked away.

I thought about my fellow resident, Jenny. Her father was a well-known surgeon in Portland. She had an altercation with a constantly rude surgical resident. She said, "John, you will never, ever get a job in Portland! I can't wait to tell my father how unprofessional and lazy you are!" Jenny was every ER resident's hero after that.

◻ ◻ ◻

Noah and I learned to windsurf in the Columbia Gorge, about an hour east of Portland. He was, annoyingly, learning faster, but I was getting the hang of it. The Columbia River forms a natural wind tunnel that passes through the towering Cascade Mountains. The Gorge cut a swath through the Cascade Range at sea level, the result of an ancient glaciated flood ripping toward the Pacific.

Under my feet, the board skipped like a stone. I gripped the sail boom until my forearms ached. I zipped back and forth across the river, navigating swell that was head high. I felt very alive.

I hit the large swell in the middle of the river and the front of the board flew up and then nosedived. I hurtled through the air and landed headfirst in the water. I swam to the surface, shook the water out of my hair, and swam back to my rig.

Noah sailed up and dropped into the water. "Nice catapult summersault."

"Thanks. I've been working on that move."

We floated in the middle of the river, resting our arms on the boards, as the sun settled in for the evening. The view was striking: backlit clouds, three-thousand-foot cliffs flanking the river, and glaciated Mount Hood in the distance.

Noah said, "You ain't in Kansas anymore, Toto."

"That's for sure. Can you believe graduation is barreling down on us? What do you think about being done? Do you feel ready?"

"I don't think you're ever ready. It's sort of like having a kid. There's never a convenient time to have children, but always a good time for practicing."

I said, "I guess we're never going be fully prepared, but it's unnerving to think about being in charge of an ER full of sick people so soon—twenty patients a day, each one depending on us.

If I think about it too long, it makes me want to spew. At least now, every decision is given the attending stamp of approval. Soon the buck will stop with us."

"And we won't be able to blame our mistakes on the boss. On the other hand, I feel much more confidant than I did a year ago."

"My confidence got rattled with that epiglottitis patient, but I guess that comes with the territory. Recently, I've felt like a cat in a room full of rocking chairs. We're signing up for a hard job. I've turned into a worrier—I'm fretting about finding a job."

"Yeah, me, too. I hate feeling so uncertain, but no matter what, next year we're going to make more money for less work."

"True. Worry never helped anything. There are several jobs available in Portland."

"Speaking of a convenient time to have children, do you and Missy have plans?"

"I think we'll wait until we've been out of residency a few years. Enjoy a little freedom. What's up with you and Suzie? You going to pop the question?"

"Wise man say: He who sticks his nose in another man's business should not be surprised to find himself with a broken nose."

"What? You asked me a personal question!"

"True, but I'm special. And this line of questioning makes me nervous. Last one to the land buys the beer." He put his feet onto his board and his hand on the boom—the wind filled his sail, pulling him out of the water—and he torpedoed toward the shore.

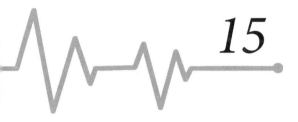

15

The long Oregon winter settled in, turning the skies into oatmeal. Time grinded like a missed gear, as I could not wait to graduate. I was killing time, and time was killing me. I was apprehensive about being done, but I was tired of residency. I wanted to spread my wings, but was scared to do so.

I tried to see as many patients as possible per shift. After graduation I would need to see every patient that shows up at the door.

I was in the middle of a busy shift, running around like a headless chicken, when the trauma pager sounded. My feet hurt and I wanted to be somewhere else.

I went to the trauma bay. The paramedics were bringing a 30-year-old stabbing victim. The patient had been stabbed in the left shoulder, and was combative in the ambulance. They would arrive in three minutes.

We began to assemble the team.

The surgical resident was Jon—I knew him pretty well; we had worked together in the surgical intensive care unit. He was a hard-working, friendly guy. He winked at me when he rushed in.

The trauma surgeon was Dr. Lowery, a no-nonsense, talented doctor. The attending emergency physician arrived, along with three nurses and a tech. We put on protective clothing: plastic face shields, gloves, and paper gowns. The tech set up the equipment for a chest tube and intubation.

We could hear the ambulance sirens approaching. The ambulance pulled in, and rapidly backed up to the open double glass doors, beeping loudly.

The rear doors of the ambulance exploded open and a paramedic burst out—drenched in sweat with his hair escaping in all directions. The patient propped on the side of the stretcher, wildly flailing and screaming curses. Another paramedic attempted to calm him.

The paramedic shouted, "We got a live wire here! He tore up the back of the ambulance. He's a heroin addict that got shanked in the neck. His name is Clark. Can you guys give us a hand?" A nurse and tech helped swing his legs up onto the stretcher.

The nurse said, "Take it easy pal, we're going to help you."

Clark said, "I'm dying! I can't breathe! Do something!" He attempted to get off the stretcher as he was wheeled to the trauma bay.

The paramedic continued, "He's been increasingly combative. He's a street guy. We haven't been able to get an IV; his veins are toast from shooting dope.

"If we knew how combative he was going to be, we would've had the police bring him. He got really wound up right before we got here. I think the only wound is at the base of his neck on the left. He wouldn't hold still for us to do much."

Clark was moved to the stretcher. He was skinny, with an acne-scarred face; his dirty hair pulled into a ponytail. His sunken eyes jumped erratically, like a dying squirrel struck by a car.

He had a look of holy terror on his face.

Droplets of bloody saliva flew from his mouth, "Help me, I'm about to die! Oh, God, I'm dying! Do something!"

I said, "Clark, hold still, we're trying to help you."

There were two people on each arm trying to start an IV. One person held while the other looked for veins. His clothes were cut and removed; he flailed naked.

Intravenous drug abusers scar their veins so it is often impossible to start an IV. Many dead-enders resort to skin-popping after they destroy their veins; they inject under the skin or into the muscle.

I studied Clark. He had one visible injury on his left shoulder, at the base of his neck, about an inch long. Dark blood flowed from the hole. Veins carry dark blood; arteries carry bright blood—rich with oxygen. The surgeons attempted to examine his neck wound but he wouldn't hold still.

Clark needed a central IV line. His deep, large veins were undamaged by his self-medication, self-mutilation. With my back to the action, I opened a central line kit. I picked up a large needle to place a central line into his femoral vein. The femoral vein is as large as a cigar and about an inch below the skin of the thigh. I attached the three-inch needle to a syringe and turned back toward Clark.

I stepped toward him, holding the syringe with both hands. He kicked my elbow and the needle sliced through the air, cutting a terrifying arc.

Jon, the surgery resident, jerked back and the stout needle barely missed his face. The needle could have pierced his flimsy plastic face shield, ripped through an eyelid, and destroyed his eye.

Everyone froze as if a pistol had fired.

Dr. Lowery ordered loudly, "Everyone step back." The troops withdrew. He continued, "Clark, stop flailing! We can't help you if you won't hold still."

Clark writhed and cursed. He cursed and writhed. He begged for help. He thrashed. Blood poured from the hole. Blood dripped off the table and onto the floor.

Dr. Lowery said to us—the team in his care, "This is unsafe. We can't approach with needles or scalpels if he is flailing. He will be still soon."

Everyone knew what he meant. When he had lost enough blood, he would stop moving.

All bleeding stops eventually.

Trauma patients are often combative. Many are drunk, high, head injured, enraged, demon-possessed, or whatever. Usually we establish an IV and manage the situation with medicines to sedate and paralyze. Then we can intubate and stabilize.

An eerie calm spread through the room. We were watching a soul die before our eyes; we did nothing. We made no eye contact. No one spoke. All eyes were on Clark as he sputtered and flung.

I felt like a witness to a medieval execution by fire—he is a drug addict and should die for his sins. Burn sinner. Burn out the demons. Burn.

I wondered about him. Who tried to murder him? Was he being robbed? Was he robbing someone? Was it revenge? How did he end up like this?

What did his mother think about how he turned out?

Did he ever know a mother's love?

What had his eyes seen?

A few minutes passed. Blood flowed out and Clark began to slow. His curses were mumbles. His movements were flickers. He was fading; his light was dimming.

He passed out.

Dr. Lowery said, "OK, let's go."

We descended. My contemplative mood transformed into action. I was wide-awake, aware. I gripped the laryngoscope and quickly passed the tube. I attached the tube to the air bag and squeezed oxygen in.

The surgery resident jammed the central line needle into his groin. Blood filled the syringe—jackpot. He connected the line to a bag of blood.

The nurse checked his blood pressure: too low.

Too low to live.

I moved to the right side of his chest to place a chest tube. I stabbed a hole between two ribs with a scalpel. I clamped the chest tube and pushed through the new wound. Blood flowed rapidly into the vacuum assisted tube.

Blood flowed out the chest tube; blood flowed in the central line—out and in, in and out.

While I was placing a chest tube, Jon approached the left side of his chest. He took a scalpel and flashed it across Clark's skin parallel to his ribs, leaving a red line. The red line fell apart, exposing glistening yellow below. He placed a rib spreader in the incision. Jon turned the crank on the spreader and the ribs parted—bursting and snapping, like a dog crunching bone.

I saw Clark's heart, the heart that held the demon that held Clark. It was still beating. Barely.

His lungs expanded with each breath squeezed in. They looked like sponges bathed in blood. Where his lung was lacerated, tiny bubbles of blood formed and popped in the maroon broth.

There was blood everywhere: dark blood, bright blood, clotted blood, still blood, swirling blood. The metallic smell of blood permeated the room, the smell of liquid iron, slightly rusty.

We frantically searched for the source of the bleeding.

Was it his heart? His aorta? His vena cava? Carotid? The jugular? Pulmonary artery?

We systematically checked. The surgeons scooped handfuls of clotted blood out. The clots landed in silver basins and plopped onto the floor like red jellyfish.

It appeared that Clark had been stabbed with a long knife in a downward motion into his chest.

His heart began to fibrillate. He had lost so much blood that the heart was now an electrical storm of malfunctioning, dying muscle: quivering instead of beating.

I grasped the two small metallic paddles used for internal electrical defibrillation—metal bars connected to four-inch disks that I placed directly on opposite sides of his vibrating heart.

I said, "Charge to ten joules! All clear? Shock!" Much less energy is needed since the paddles were placed directly on the heart.

Shock.

His heart jolted and began to beat again.

The two surgeons re-entered the chest with their hands as fast as I could get the paddles out.

Jon said, "I think he's bleeding from the arch of his subclavian vein. Clamp."

The nurse slapped a clamp into his hand. He reached in and placed a clamp on one side of the large bleeding vein.

"Another clamp." Smack.

He frantically suctioned blood, "I can't see anything in here!"

Dr. Lowery replied, "Just take your time, you're almost there."

Jon said, "Three-oh nylon stitch on a large needle driver."

He tied off the bleeding vessel. Blood continued to fill the chest, a leaky boat filling with dark water—evil dark water.

Jon said, "There must be another bleeder. Where is it?"

He was soaked in sweat and splattered with blood. He turned to a nurse who wiped his face shield with a damp cloth.

Clark's heart began to have another seizure, vibrating chaotically.

I grabbed the paddles and re-entered his chest. I could feel his heart vibrating through the metal in my hands. "Twenty joules!"

Shock.

Nothing.

"Thirty joules!"

"Forty!" The heart shook with each shock, but so does a dead horse when kicked.

"Again."

"Again." I reached in, grasped the heart, and squeezed it rhythmically: CPR on an open chest. I held the possessed heart and squeezed and squeezed and squeezed but the demons had been in there for too long—too much evil, too much destruction.

Clark's face was whitewashed like a peppermint sucked of the color; the color had spilled all over the floor. We were unable to keep up; the color was sucked from his body faster than we could replace it.

I knew it was hopeless; Clark was dead. We gave him cardiac medicines and worked a few more minutes, but they had won. We lost. The devil, the demons, and Clark's murderer had won.

We stopped the open cardiac massage and declared him dead about one hour after he arrived in the ER.

I went to see new patients and finish the ones I had already started on. Jon left to finish rounding on his patients on the floor. We all went back to what we were doing, business as usual.

◘ ◘ ◘

After my shift, I was in the locker room, changing out of my scrubs. Franklin walked in. We were alone. I was not in the mood.

"Hey, Brent, what's up, buddy?"

"Nothing." Buddy.

"You headed back to the South after graduation?" He spoke with an exaggerated, mocking, fake Southern accent.

"No." I simmered. I noticed Clark's blood on my shoe.

He feigned surprise, "Oh. Where do you want to work?"

"Hopefully, here in Portland."

"Oh. Wow. Hmmm." An awkward pause, "I thought you were going back to the South."

You thought wrong, ding-dong. "No. We like it here."

"Noah's going back to old Miss?"

"He's from Georgia, but he wants to stay here."

He raised his eyebrows—concerned. "I didn't know you guys wanted to stay here. I keep my finger on the pulse of the job market. I have contacts in most of the ERs around town...."

Sure you do.

"And I haven't heard either of you mentioned as candidates. Have you applied?"

"Yes." I buttoned my shirt.

"Have you sent in a formal resume? That's important. They want to know where you went to college..."

You: Yale. Me: Mississippi State.

"and your research and publications..."

None.

"honor societies and..."

I interrupted, "I've sent my resume to a few hospitals."

With mock relief he said, "So you've applied. Have you heard anything?"

"No." I tied my shoe.

"No offers? None?"

I said nothing.

He said, "Just deafening silence, huh?"

I stood and gazed at him, "Have a good shift, Franklin." I turned and walked out.

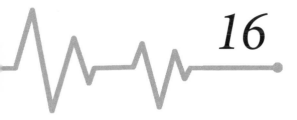

16

The hole was enormous. I had been here before, but every time I was blown away by the magnitude. I looked at Noah standing on the lip; the yawning abyss open at his feet. The sun reflected off of the snow. We could see Mount Rainier, Mount Adams, Mount Hood, and the Columbia River Gorge in the distance. Each volcano was perfectly snow capped. The crater on Mount Saint Helens is about one and half miles in diameter and over two thousand feet deep. Volcanic steam rose from the crater; the pungent sulfur stung my nose as I stared into the giant mouth—the mouth that once spat half a mountain across a pristine mountain landscape: a spitting Saint.

I imagined what the eruption was like, on that fateful day in 1980 when a zillion tons of debris—heated far beyond the melting point of rock—hurtled across the landscape at hundreds of miles an hour, possibly faster than the speed of sound. I could see downed trees—giant burnt matches—in the blast zone. The thermal energy released was over 1500 times the size of the atomic bomb dropped on Hiroshima. I felt small.

We ate lunch and I told Noah about Clark. I said, "It was odd. After he died in front of our eyes, I didn't feel much. I didn't feel sad or helpless or anything."

"Yeah, I don't feel much, usually."

"Do you think we're being robbed of our humanity?"

He said, "What's the other option? Go cry about it? Take it home with you and ruin your life?"

"I have a vague worry that we're turning into robots."

"I think being a bit robotic is probably a good thing, R2D2. We're providing care to the most injured patients and trying to stay sane. The ability to be clinical is our salvation. The people who make it in this job are the ones who can compartmentalize."

"True. We know a few mentally unhealthy doctors."

"That's for sure."

"Everyone has their neuroses, but I suspect the majority of mentally-tilted doctors suffer from a combination of their inability to compartmentalize, arrogance, and power tripping. And some stayed in from recess to avoid sports and bullies."

He said, "The Revenge of the Nerds. Aren't some of those guys freaks? Freaks! I was in surgery with a cardiac surgeon with a pathological ego. I had the grunt med student job, holding the skin with tweezers while he cut. He said, 'You are holding the skin too firmly! How would you like someone to pinch your skin like that? Hold out your hand!'

"I held out my hand. He took a hemostat and pinched my gloved hand in the web space between my thumb and index finger. It broke the glove and my skin! It hurt like sin! With a bloody instrument he was using for surgery!"

I said, "Holy Moses! What did you do?"

"Nothing. I suppose if I had made a stink about it, he would have gotten in trouble, but he was one of the most prominent surgeons in the region and big business for the hospital."

I said, "I know the most bizarre doctor on the earth's face." I proceeded to tell Noah about a trauma surgeon from my med school.

⊞ ⊞ ⊞

Dr. Syke, affectionately called Dr. Psycho by the residents, was a spectacular—but severely egotistic—surgeon. If it was possible to heal someone by slicing, Psycho could do it. If it were possible to maintain order in the chaos of the ER, he could do it. He was a perfectionist who rose to the occasion when it hit the fan. He had wild mood swings; when he was in a dark place he was somewhat of a sadist. He had a reputation for wild living—late nights and early mornings.

He was the champion of berating residents; Dr. Psycho loved to ask questions until he found an unknown, and then make you feel like an imbecile.

He asked me what a patient's blood count was; when I glanced at my notes, he tore into me like a tornado in a trailer park. He snarled, "On the surgery floor, we expect our med students to come to rounds prepared. What is your problem, boy?"

He had a tyrannical personality that was so clichéd, it was comical. He often spoke of his grandiose accomplishments, including his triple black belt in karate. He was an avid hunter; he often traveled to Africa on big game hunts. He drove a Ferrari and always had a loaded pistol on his person. He had a gizmo in his car that popped a gun up from underneath the seat when he pushed a button on the steering wheel, ostensibly to protect him from carjackers. He maintained that he needed to be locked and loaded at all times to protect himself from rival gang members—many of his patients were injured in gang-related violence.

And a meteor might land on your head, Dr. Psycho. It could happen. You can never be too careful. Maybe you should wear a helmet walking down the street.

He loved to rush into the ER when a trauma alert was paged, setting off metal detectors with his pistol—Superman coming to save the day! I secretly wished for a meteor of Kryptonite.

I remember Dr. Psycho bursting through the ambulance bay doors, setting off the metal alarm. He turned toward the security guard and slapped the side of his chest, demonstrating his chest holster and his piece—a man's man, packing heat. The security guard appeared to appreciate his manliness. Psycho's eyes danced wildly with anticipation of the battle.

Dr. Psycho spoke loudly to a resident, "Did I tell you about the polar bear I bagged last week? I went on a hunting trip to the Northern Territories and got a real trophy. I'm going to have her mounted and put in my entry foyer."

I thought, like we care about your hunting, Psycho. Or your guns or your karate—just shut up and do your job.

Once he told a joke on rounds, "I collect guns, but I don't shoot people with them. Just cans. Like Afri-cans. Mexi-cans, Puerto Ri-cans."

As much as he irritated me, I had to admit that he was the best; nobody could run a trauma like Psycho. His skills in the operating room were legendary.

After I moved to Oregon, I spoke with one of my buddies from med school and he told me what happened with Psycho after I left Birmingham.

The ER got a call from the paramedics about a severely injured 48-year-old; he was in a motorcycle accident and had multiple injuries. He was intubated. His chest was caved in. He had multiple orthopedic fractures.

The trauma attending for the week was Dr. Bizovi, the chief of surgery and one of two remaining board-certified trauma surgeons at the University. There had been a recent exodus of the trauma surgeons on staff and the University had been trying to hire more. Dr. Bizovi and Dr. Psycho had been on call every other week: a brutal schedule.

The ambulance turned in and a back door opened. The paramedic jumped out and rushed in. He said, "It's Dr. Syke, the surgeon!" Dr. Psycho.

The room was filled with dread. Everyone was still; all of the oxygen had been sucked from the room, like a backdraft in a house fire.

The ambulance doors blew open and oxygen was added to the smoldering backdraft; the room exploded into action. The paramedics rolled Dr. Psycho into the bay, his bloody mouth agape, the endotracheal tube hanging like a giant fish hook. His intense eyes were swollen shut. His leather motorcycle gear was abraded and torn. Every member of the team descended on him—cutting off his clothes and assessing injuries.

The medic said that Dr. Psycho was involved in a motorcycle crash traveling at a high rate of speed on the interstate. Witnesses said that he hit a guardrail and flipped through the air. He landed on pavement and slid into rocks on the side of the road. He had a fractured left femur and right humerus. His left leg was bent at the thigh and his lower leg was folded behind his back; the fracture was open. He was unconscious. His helmet was crushed.

Dr. Bizovi moved in and placed his hands on his partner. The trauma surgeons tend to stand back and direct from afar, letting the residents do most of the procedures. Not with this patient.

He was wearing a chest holster, and his ribs were crushed where the gun had been trapped between the pavement and the doctor. There was a open wound into his chest cavity that sucked air every time he took a breath—Psycho could still suck the air out of a room.

Dr. Bizovi took a scalpel and cut into his friend's chest. I don't know if Psycho had any real friends, but those two men had worked together for almost twenty years.

Dr. Psycho was horribly injured. He had multiple fractures, a terrible chest wound, and his liver was lacerated.

One of the two trauma surgeons at the University was a trauma patient. He was sliced open by a team of residents that he had probably browbeaten the week before. His partner, Dr. Bizovi, struggled to keep him out of the Happy Hunting Grounds—just as Psycho had done with many souls in the past.

Dr. Psycho survived. He spent months in the hospital and eventually recovered.

◫　◫　◫

Noah picked up a snowball and tossed it absentmindedly down the snowy slopes. He said, "What a freakshow! Doctors can be some of the weirdest people."

I said, "Some are driven to succeed because they have something to prove. An ego that feeds on the adoration of others creates instability—those types can be such divas. Fame and fortune ain't good for the soul."

I clicked on my skis and Noah strapped on his snowboard. It had taken us about five hours to hike up in the snow.

Changing the subject to something more pleasant and worthy of the surroundings, he said, "I love the smell of melting snow mixed with fir trees. Check out Spirit Lake down there." He pointed at the once-pristine lake that had sloshed eight hundred feet up the slopes of the Saint, now full of downed trees from the eruption.

I said, "I could stay here a week. We should do that next year when we have more free time. We could camp for a few days. I've camped with my brother here."

"Did you know Saint Helen is the patron saint of divorced people and difficult marriages?"

He made the sign of the cross over my chest, blessing me. He quickly shoved me backwards against the slope. I fell onto my seat. He laughed and said, "I'll race you down!" He barreled down the slopes of the Saint with wings of flying snow following him; like an angel on fire, screaming toward a lake of holy water.

MIRACLES and MAYHEM in the ER

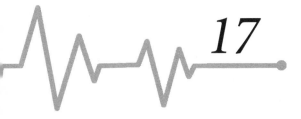

We were at a Portland Trailblazers basketball game with our better halves. Ricky and Noah followed the team religiously. A few years later, one of the star players, Travis Outlaw, came from my high school in Mississippi. Several of my high school teammates were his cousins and they came to Portland to watch him play. I knew some of his family from Fred's church. It's a small world, after all.

Ricky brought us popcorn and leaned over and kissed his wife, Paula. Paula was surprisingly attractive. She reminded me of a country music singer. Ricky had been on a roll, telling new people his old stories.

Ricky said, "I told Paula it seemed like 'A Weekend at Bernie's.' You seen that movie? They carry around a dead guy and act like he's alive, just like those EMTs with the man who choked on the steak."

Noah said, "Just when I think I've heard them all."

Ricky said, "Your pal, Franklin Trader, is doing his EMS rotation now. I see why you guys complain about him. None of the paramedics can stand him. He got one of my buddies in trouble for going home during a shift. They went to his house to watch television during a lull. Franklin went with him, then blabbed about it to our boss!"

Noah said, "Sounds about right."

I said, "I've given up on trying to understand that guy. He probably was trying to cover himself if somehow there was trouble.

He's paranoid; no one from our residency would care if he watched TV during a lull on his EMS rotation."

Ricky said, "He tries to make us feel stupid. He asks questions like, 'If this turns out to be pseudomonas pneumonia, what would be our antibiotic choices?' Like we're going to know the answer to that."

I said, "That sounds like Dr. Psycho from med school. He always asked questions we couldn't answer to feel superior."

Ricky said, "Well, just like Dr. Psycho, we gave Dr. Trader a nickname—Dr. Traitor."

Noah said, "Dr. Traitor! I like it!" Missy and I laughed.

Paula said, "Ricky! Be nice!"

"Sorry, sweetie. "

Suzie said, "Noah, tell Brent what you heard Franklin say."

Noah shot her a look and said, "Let's talk about a more pleasant topic. Did you guys get ski passes?"

Ricky said, "Skiing is for people who can see their own shoes."

An hour later, I followed Noah to the restroom. "What was Suzie talking about?"

"Don't worry about it. Just Franklin being an idiot."

"You know I'm going to bug you until you tell me."

"He was talking to Brad Williams about job prospects." Brad was a recent grad from our residency. He worked at a nice community hospital. "Brad was discussing potential job openings in Portland. Franklin said that he thought most people would be looking for jobs in Portland, except you. He told Brad about the shoulder dislocation and the epiglottitis cases."

I was stunned. It felt like I had been punched in the nose and was seeing white spots. I immediately started thinking about finding him and letting him have it with both barrels. My jaw tensed and my teeth grinded like a power sander.

For him to trash my job prospects was an act of reckless violence that I would make him account for. I would make him pay. He had gone too far this time. He would pay.

I muttered, "I'm going to kill him."

"Don't worry about it; I took up for you. I said that you had great evaluations and don't make any more mistakes than the rest of us. Brad's smart enough to see through his crap."

I seethed, "Maybe. But he's making both of us look stupid. I'm going to confront him and it isn't going to be pretty."

"I can see why you are angry. I was also, but I don't think confronting him is the best play. Better to ignore him. The bigger deal you make, the worse it'll be. That's why I wasn't going to tell you about it. I knew you'd get riled up."

"But sometimes you have to punch a bully in the nose." I relished the thought.

"True, sometimes you do. But fighting him will be like fighting the tar baby; the more you punch the more mired you'll get. What does he have to lose? He already has a smarmy reputation. Just let him be. Brad knows you're a good doctor and he probably knows Franklin is a jerk. Frankie looked fairly stupid when I contradicted him."

I returned to my seat in a foul mood and watched the game, sulking. Missy asked me what was wrong. I stared straight ahead and said, "Nothing."

By the end of the game, I was feeling better, but I didn't know what I was going to do when I saw Dr. Traitor. Noah was right, better to ignore him. I was not sure if I could.

After the game, we walked to a pub. I was in a better mood—I was with some of my favorite people.

Noah asked, "Ricky, have you told Brent about that guy who should win a Darwin award? The one you took care of in eastern Oregon?"

"I don't think so. That one's the doozy of all doozies! You ain't gonna believe the behavior of these dudes. Lordamighty!"

We leaned in to hear. Ricky told a lot of stories, but he never told boring stories.

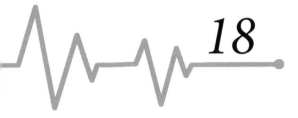

18

Ricky was working in rural eastern Oregon—a small cowboy town mostly inhabited by ranchers and farmers. He worked as a tech in the ER and a paramedic when there were ambulance calls.

He heard the ambulance radio crackle. "We have a critically injured person—someone shot, bitten and then electrocuted in a bathtub. The caller said the man is nearly dead."

Ricky picked up the radio for more details. The dispatcher said, "The patient is in a bathtub on Ice Creek Road. The caller wouldn't identify himself but the call was made from the same address."

Ricky and his partner fired up the lights and sirens. After driving about fifteen miles through the high desert sagebrush, they pulled up to a ramshackle mobile home with random debris in the front yard: a lawnmower engine, a rusted baby crib, a partially melted artificial Christmas tree resting in a patch of burnt grass, and a huge satellite dish tipped on its side. There were two pickup trucks in the driveway. There were no other houses for a quarter of a mile.

When they pulled into the drive, Ricky muttered to Tommy, his partner, "Wait a minute. Chill Coyote lives here."

"What kind of name is that?"

"He's as strange as they get."

A light inside went out; he saw someone peer out a window and then quickly pull the blind. Ricky had an uneasy feeling.

They unloaded the stretcher and rolled it toward the front door, stepping over black plastic bags full of garbage. Several looked like an animal had torn into them; garbage was strewn about. Ricky avoided stepping on eggshells and his foot smeared dog feces. He rapped on the door.

No answer. He knocked again. No answer.

Ricky said loudly, "We're the paramedics! We're here about the accident victim!"

Silence.

He yelled, "Look, we know someone's in there! Open the door or we'll call the Sheriff! I know who lives here, so get out here and talk to me! Now!"

A voice from inside said, "OK, I'm coming! Is that you, Ritchie?" Ricky rolled his eyes.

A man in his mid-thirties opened the door. He had an out-turned eye, tattooed arms, and random teeth. He looked like something that had been pulled from a garbage can. He said, "Can't a man take a nap in peace? What do you want?" He stepped out and closed the door behind.

"We got a call from this house that there was a critically ill patient here with multiple injuries."

Coyote ran his fingers through his greasy hair and feigned surprise, "Here? You guys must have the wrong address. There's no one here but me. There's nobody hurt here." He studied at his arms as if inspecting for injuries, first his palms and then the back of his hands and arms. He looked up with eyebrows raised.

A loud crash came from inside the house.

Ricky said, "What was that, Coyote?"

"Uh, probably my dog."

"Can we come in and look around?"

"What for?"

"Because we got a call that there's someone practically dead here. You're acting fishy."

"Fishy? What're you talking about, Ritchie? I just want to go back to sleep. I was taking a nap." He faked a yawn.

"Can we come in and look around?"

"Do you have a search warrant?"

Ricky snapped, "Why would we have a search warrant? We came to help a wounded person, not to arrest anyone. I'm sure I could get a sheriff here without much effort."

"O.K., come in then. But, there ain't nobody hurt here."

Coyote yelled, "Guys, the ambulance dudes are coming in. For some crazy reason they think someone is hurt here. I told them there wasn't."

They heard sounds of feet pounding the hollow trailer, and then water running. Someone yelled, "Come on in, we're just watching TV."

They left the stretcher outside, and walked into a cramped den with a naked light bulb observing the scene like an eye. The room was decorated with a faded poster of a woman in a bikini lying on the hood of a Ferrari, all four appendages spread eagle, lipstick leering at the camera. Another poster caged a devilish skull with flames coming out of the sockets. Two mangy looking humans were sitting on a bile-green couch, held together by stains.

One of them stood and extended his damp hand, "I'm Hacksaw and this is Buzzsaw." He was missing one front tooth, the other was loose and wobbled when he spoke. The periphery of his face was smeared with a reddish material; his T-shirt was wet on the shoulders.

Ricky said, "You guys like watching the TV with it turned off?"

Hacksaw said, "Oh, yeah. We was just about to turn it on. Anything you want to watch?"

Ricky said, "Why do you have blood on your face?"

"I cut myself shaving."

"That's just ketchup."

"Which is it, guys?"

"Ketchup." "Shaving accident." Spoken simultaneously.

Ricky said, "Look fellas, it's obvious something is wrong here. If you don't cooperate, I'll be forced to call the sheriff."

Coyote interjected, "O.K., we're sorry. We accidentally called 911 because we were trying to prank call a friend. Hacksaw cut himself shaving and we thought it'd be funny to have our friend come over and see the blood and think he was really hurt."

Ricky said, "Where are you cut, Hacksaw? You would've had to cut off your nose to bleed that much. It's all over you." He pointed at Buzz, "Look at Buzz, he has it all over his clothes."

Coyote continued, "That's fake blood. We put that on them to make it seem worse." His two friends nodded their heads vigorously in agreement.

Ricky said, "May I look into the other rooms? We'll leave you alone after that."

"Uh, sure. You won't tell the sheriff if there's any sort of illegal stuff, will you?"

"As long as we don't find any dead bodies or child porno."

The three men burst out laughing: terribly acted, fake laughing. All mouths were open and their horrible teeth were on full display. Hacksaw looked like a clown ghoul with his bloody face, sunken eyes, and solitary fang.

Ricky and Tommy stared steely eyed at them while they awkwardly hee-hawed for entirely too long.

They moved through the house. Every room was strewn with dirty clothes and stinking food; beer cans were littered about. When they walked into the kitchen, a glass marijuana bong sat on the kitchen table. Buzzsaw tossed a dirty towel over it, knocking it over. It rolled off the table and crashed on the floor, shattering glass and spilling water. Hacksaw glared at Buzzsaw and began to speak. He stopped and quickly smiled.

Nothing to see here people, just keep moving.

No one said anything. Tommy and Ricky smirked at each other.

After they looked around enough to be convinced there were no mortally wounded people in the trailer, they walked outside.

Coyote followed. "Sorry you good fellas had to come out on account of our foolishness. We didn't mean to call 911. We're real sorry. For real. For rizzle." A toothy smile.

Ricky said, "Stay out of trouble, Coyote."

They got into the ambulance. Ricky said, "There's something wrong, but what in the world?"

Tommy said, "Those guys seem like real gems."

Ricky said, "Local lowlifes."

Tommy asked, "What about those names?"

"They gave themselves those nicknames long ago. I guess they thought it'd help them communicate under the radar with their illicit activities, first with teachers and later police. What a bunch of Howdy-Doodys!"

"What should we do? Should we call the sheriff? It seems that they are up to no good, but I don't want to rat on them if they're just smoking a little weed."

Tommy said, "I suppose it's possible that they got injured in some way and were high and confused and called 911. We shouldn't get them into trouble."

Ricky said, "But what if they murdered someone? Or tried to murder someone? There could be a body in the woods behind their house, or under the trailer. We should call the sheriff."

"Yeah, you're right. They have to know a sheriff will be out there soon. If they have a lick of sense—which is far from certain—they will have cleaned up their bong and weed."

Ricky laughed, "What bong? That thing shattered like my ex-girlfriend's heart!"

They talked with the sheriff and went back to the ER. About an hour later the sheriff called and spoke with Ricky.

Ricky told Tommy, "The sheriff has a warrant for all three of those geeks for parole violations. They've each spent time in jail for petty crime. He said that when he went to the house, there were no cars out front; they must've left. The house is a rental. He's going to get a search warrant and search the house."

They waited.

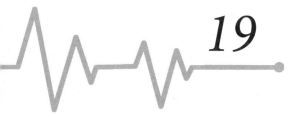

19

A few hours later they got a different call. Ricky took the call and said, "A panicked woman says there's a man at her house, nearly dead. She got home after work and found a naked guy in her bathtub. The tub's full of blood and ice. Let's rumble!" Tommy and Ricky ran to the ambulance.

Ricky said, "What do you think? Homicide or suicide? Most people that cut their wrists to commit suicide do it in warm water, not ice. Warm water prevents clotting."

"Maybe it was someone who got their kidneys stolen by organ robbers."

"I'm pretty sure that's a hoax or an urban legend. I don't think that's ever happened, at least not in the U.S."

"This is BFE, Oregon. Who said it was the U.S.?"

Ricky smiled, "True. This is the frontier, any farther and we fall off the edge. The address is just about a mile from where we were earlier."

"Do you think this is related?"

"We don't get called for bleeding, severely injured people but about once a month. Nearly-dead, naked people in bathtubs are slightly more rare."

Tommy laughed, "You never know. Sometimes I will see ten naked people in bathtubs a night. Almost as common as the cold."

Ricky said, "This town is full of people you'd expect if Little House on the Prairie bred with zombies."

They arrived. It was also a mobile home. The front yard was well kept. There were a few ceramic statues and a concrete birdfeeder in the freshly cut patch of grass. There was a sign on the front door: "God Bless This Home."

The door burst open; a broad homely woman bustled out. "Oh, thank God that you're here! Freak Dog is practically dead in my bathtub."

Ricky said, "What happened?"

"I don't know. I came home from work and there was blood all over my front door. I was scared to go in, but against all better knowing, I went inside. I heard a moaning from my bathroom, and I found Freak Dog sitting in the bathtub full of bloody ice, naked as the day he was born. He can't say what happened. He's totally out of it."

They quickly went inside. They parked the stretcher next to the omnipresent modern idol—the glass faced box on a gilded stand—wires and antennae bringing the idol to life daily for limitless adoration and worship.

They moved down the tight hall decorated with family photos and a print of a tropical beach at sunset. They found Freak Dog in the tub.

Tommy grabbed his feet and Ricky his upper body. Their rubber gloves had difficulty gripping his slippery ankles. Blush-colored water dripped onto their scrubs as they sloshed him out of the tub. Ice clattered and moved rapidly across the linoleum.

They struggled with his wet bloody body down the narrow hall into the cramped living room where they heaved him onto the stretcher. His hand smeared the television—a blood offering to the idol.

Tommy asked, "Do you have any clue what happened? Has he been suicidal? Could this be a murder attempt?"

She replied, "I doubt either one. He's not really what you'd call a law-abiding citizen, but I don't think anyone would want to kill him. He usually seems pretty happy."

Ricky asked, "How do you know him?"

"I date his friend, Earl. Most folks call him Buzzsaw." At least she picked the one with all his teeth.

Tommy said, "Can you come with us to the hospital? The more information, the better."

"Sure. I'll follow you to the hospital in my car."

They loaded Freak Dog into the ambulance and fired the sirens.

Tommy asked, "What do you think?"

Ricky replied, "I got no idea. This is the weirdest thing I've seen in my entire life. I knew those clowns were up to something."

Ricky examined Freak. He was breathing but incoherent, moaning softly. He had multiple tattoos of snakes and dragons; one across his chest said, "Inbred Pot Head." The hypothermia and smeared blood created a pattern as though finger painted with crimson streaks over his polar blue skin.

He had strange injuries all over his body—a riddle of wounds. Ricky checked his blood pressure: very low. His temperature was eighty-nine degrees. He had been in the ice water for quite some time, floating above the drain.

He was circling the drain.

Tommy shouted over the siren, "What did the first caller say? That he'd been electrocuted?"

Ricky said, "Shot, electrocuted, and bitten. I bet this wound on his right thigh is a gunshot." He studied the half-inch hole above his knee where dark blood was oozing. The left calf had two charred areas surrounded by large purple blisters, weeping clear fluid. "Maybe this charred area is where he was electrocuted. There're a couple of knife wounds here. This was an attempted homicide."

Tommy said, "Did you look at his back to see if his kidneys have been removed?"

"Sorry, there's nothing on his back. Nice try."

"Dang it, I was hoping to be on CNN!"

Ricky said, "It looks like he was tortured with electricity and a knife. I bet this was a drug deal that went off the rails."

Ricky started an IV and hung fluids. They pulled into the ambulance bay at the ER. The nurses and doctor were waiting.

The doc said, "Can you bring warming blankets and warm IV fluid? We need a second IV. Send blood; order blood for transfusion. He appears to have lost a lot.

"Bring the intubation equipment. I'm hopeful he might turn around with warming and IV fluids. I wish I could talk with him to find out what happened. If he hasn't perked up in thirty minutes or so, I will intubate him for transport. Call the transport helicopter. We're going to transfer him ASAP." They continued the resuscitation.

Buzzsaw's girlfriend, Janet, arrived. "How's he doing? Is he going to live?"

Ricky said, "I'm not sure, but I think so. We need to know what happened to him to treat him appropriately. Earlier, we were called to a different address and your boyfriend and two other men were there. They were covered in blood and told us they had accidentally called 911."

"Was it Earl, Hacksaw, and Chill Coyote?"

Tommy interjected, "Yes; that's exactly who it was. They lied to us. What is going on?"

"I have no idea. Those four spend lots of time together; none of them have a real job. Earl told me last night that they were going to scout for elk today. That usually means that they'll sit around in their pickups in a field, drinking beer and smoking weed."

Ricky said, "Someone tortured and tried to murder him."

"I don't know who'd do such a thing. They just hang out with each other. They aren't involved in any serious criminal things; I'm almost positive. They don't do hard drugs anymore. None of those guys would hurt anyone."

Ricky said, "Can you ask your boyfriend to come? I won't call the sheriff if he'll come in. If he doesn't, they're going to be hunted. They'll be the primary suspects in this crime."

"I'll call him on his cell. You promise not to call the cops?"

"Promise."

A few minutes later she returned. "They're coming. They want to meet you and the doc in the parking lot."

They went to check on Freak. He mumbled a few words. His blood pressure was better and his temperature was rising.

The doc said, "The copter will be in the air shortly. It should be here in less than thirty minutes."

Freak's tests showed severe blood loss and kidney damage. An X-ray showed a bullet lodged in his femur.

A few minutes later, Ricky and Tommy walked in with Coyote, Buzzsaw, and Hacksaw. He turned to them and said, "You have a lot of explaining to do. Start talking."

They glanced around nervously. Coyote began, "We was hanging out in the countryside, listening to music, talking and drinking. Freak had gotten pretty twisted. A big snake slithered through the sagebrush—huge—big around as my arm. Freak said he was a snake charmer and he's going to kill the snake. He got his axe handle out of his truck. He keeps it under the seat in case of he needs to mete out some justice."

Hack interjected, "He ain't never used it though."

"I'm telling this story! The man is sick and we don't need you interrupting!" He paused and glared at Hack, "Anyway, he got the axe handle and went to whack the snake. The snake coiled up, and that rattle shook."

Hack said, "It sounded like dried beans in a bowl."

Coyote closed his eyes and bowed his head, slowly shaking it side to side, as if valiantly trying to contain his last patient nerve. He continued, "As he walked toward it, the snake sprung and struck him in the leg below the knee, and then wrapped around his leg. Freak jumped around, screaming. It was probably four to five feet long. He beat at it until it let go and slithered off."

Ricky snapped, "What about his other injuries? Why was he in tub full of ice?"

"I'm getting to that." He paused and frowned at Ricky. Ricky frowned back harder, and threw up his hands.

He continued, "So, anyway, then he cussed and screamed and rolled around on the ground for a bit. We told him he needed to go to the hospital. He said he wanted revenge and ain't no snake going to get away with biting him. He said that his daddy taught him to be a snake charmer when he was a little boy."

Hack's abominable teeth escaped from their oral cage into a dreadful smile, "He always says his daddy taught him this or that, like he's the expert on everything."

"Shut up! Please! Do you want to tell the story?" Coyote scowled at Hack, who—in turn—studied his shoelaces.

Coyote continued, "So he gimped to his truck and got out his pistol. He named his pistol Cop Killa, even though I'm pretty sure all his dealings with police involve him begging and whining."

Ricky said, "You don't need to tell all about his life. The doc needs to know what happened to him."

"If everyone quits interrupting, I could tell the story." He crossed his arms and looked away: a pouting child.

The doc turned to Buzz, who seemed to have stage fright. He looked at Hack.

Hack said, "Freak walked over with his gun to shoot the rattler and when he shot at it, the bullet ricocheted off a rock and hit him in his other leg. He flipped around in the dirt. He couldn't walk since both legs was messed up.

"I knew that you're supposed to cut the bite open and suck the poison out, so I cut his leg with my pocketknife. He screamed when I cut him, but I knew it was for his good. I sucked blood and spit it out. When I asked these guys to take a turn, they just stared. Didn't even help."

Coyote said, "Because it was disgusting and nasty. You looked like a jungle cannibal, with blood all around your mouth, and everyone knows that don't work. I knew electricity was the way to neutralize the poison; I remembered that from health class. That's right, huh, doc?"

The doctor said, "Keep going."

He said, "I hooked the jumper cables to the truck battery. We held him down and put the clamps on each side of the wound by pinching his skin. We fired up the engine and he rolled around screaming until he knocked the clamps off. His skin got cooked and smelled like burnt meat, but I'm sure we neutralized some of the poison."

Ricky asked, "Why didn't you just bring him into the ER? That would've been better."

Coyote didn't reply. Buzz and Hack looked like middle-schoolers caught with cigarettes.

Ricky said, "You guys better start talking or there are going to be problems!"

Coyote said slowly, "Are you saying electricity don't work?"

The doc said, "No, it doesn't work and neither does sucking blood. Why didn't you just bring him in?"

No answer.

Ricky said, "Answer him!"

Coyote looked chastened, "We have outstanding warrants. We was afraid someone would call the cops. You guys promised not to call the cops, right?"

The doctor said, "What happened next?"

Coyote said, "He was pretty out of it, and his leg was bleeding where he'd gotten shot. Hack had heard that cold water helps blood to clot. Is that true?"

"Sort of. It helps clot blood and slow down circulation, but…" He paused, and said, "Just keep going."

"We went to Buzzsaw's girlfriend's house and put him in the bathtub. We got some ice at the gas station and iced him down. He started looking like he might die or something, so we came up with a plan to leave him and call 911 and tell where he was. That way we wouldn't all have to go to jail, and we figured Freak Dog would rather be in jail than dead."

"Why did you give the wrong address?"

Hack said, "Cause Coyote's an idiot and gave the wrong address. He gave the address of the house where he lives instead of Janet's address."

"At least I didn't go slobbering in the wound like Count Chocula. And, I have both my front teeth."

Hack retorted, "It's Dracula, stupid! At least I don't have an eye that looks sideways. Helloooo? Are you looking at me?" He waved his hand back and forth in front of Coyote's face.

A nurse interrupted, "The patient is talking. I think he's getting better. The blood's here, do you want me to hang it?"

"Yeah, he needs the blood."

The sheriff pulled up outside; they could see his car through the glass ambulance bay doors. Coyote, Hacksaw, and Buzzsaw looked petrified.

Coyote said, "Aw, Ricky, how could you? You betrayed us!"

"I didn't call him. He probably heard from the 911 operator when your girlfriend called."

Coyote looked like he was about to cry, "I can't stand the thought of another year in the big house. I don't think I can take it."

Ricky said softly, "If you walk out that door, I'll talk with him and buy you time. I'm not going to lie, but I may be able to stall him."

His eyes lit up and Coyote whispered, "Thanks dude. We owe you!"

They hurried out. The sheriff was still inside the squad car. The dome light was on and he was writing.

The doc and Ricky walked into Freak's room; he was more alert. He groaned, "What happened?"

The doctor explained the situation and said, "We're going to transfer you by helicopter. The copter should be here in less than ten minutes. You'll receive antivenom to counteract the snake's venom. We don't have antivenom here. You'll need surgery on the bullet wound. You may need skin grafting where you were bitten and burnt."

"Don't worry about me; my daddy taught me how to make it in situations like this."

Ricky thought, Situations like what? Snake bitten, shot, stabbed, electrocuted, frozen situations?

The doc said, "You'll receive very good care."

"I'm a survivor; I'll survive."

⬚ ⬚ ⬚

I shook my head in disbelief.

Suzie asked, "What happened to them?"

Ricky took a sip of beer and said, "Freak escaped the hospital a day early and no one heard from them for a long time. The sheriff was not too concerned with rounding them up.

"I saw them once or twice afterward. Freak lost some muscle in his leg, but was able to walk pretty good. I don't think they ever went to jail.

"The entire town was abuzz with the story of the gaggle of idiots. They probably laid low due to embarrassment as much as anything."

Noah raised his bottle, "This one is to Chainsaw, Buzz Freak, Chilly Dog, Snake Whatever and, most of all, to my man—Quick Ricky!"

Ricky laughed, "I'm not sure I want to be lumped into that crowd."

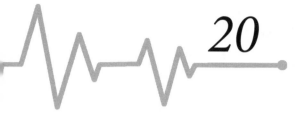

20

The brain colored clouds started to break up and the blue skies were making a comeback. Spring popped with bloom, and I marked the days. Missy made a paper chain and we tore off a link daily, anticipating graduation. I could not wait to be done, even though residency was a generally positive experience, and I had trepidation about being on my own.

I saw the light at the end of the tunnel. So close.

I was working a shift at the University. I picked up the next chart. The complaint was listed as "I have something in my ear."" I walked into the room and met the patient—a professional middle-aged woman. She said, "I feel something scratching inside my ear."

"When did you notice it?"

"Yesterday. It feels like something is moving in there."

"Let's have a look." I peered into her ear with an otoscope. There was a complete spider web with a tiny spider right in the middle, fully suspended in her ear canal. It looked like a microscopic version of Charlotte's Web.

I said, "You're not going to believe this, but you have a spider in your ear."

She looked mortified, "You're kidding right? A spider? Really?"

"Yeah, it's a complete spider web with a spider." I drew her a picture: a few concentric circles with a spider on the bull's eye.

She looked like she would rather have inoperable brain cancer, or permanent uncontrollable diarrhea. Her upper lip perspired; she whispered, "What are you going to do?"

143

"It'll be easy." I took a long Q-tip; I smashed the tiny spider and pulled it out of her ear.

She said, "I have to go home and lie down."

▣　▣　▣

I heard vomiting from a patient's room. I walked over to see if I could assist. I saw a resident doctor vomiting repetitively into the trashcan. The patient was lying on his side, facing away from the doctor. The resident looked at me and wiped his mouth. With tears in his eyes, he said softly, "I'm all right. I'm draining an abscess." The stench of the abscess was overwhelming. I walked out of the room without saying anything.

A few minutes later, he emerged from the room. I asked, "Are you sick? Do you need to go home?"

He said, "No, I'm not sick. I couldn't stand the smell. That's the worst abscess I've ever drained."

▣　▣　▣

My patient was a 20-year-old woman who told the triage nurse, "I'm going to kill myself! I can't go on! My boyfriend broke up with me!" She threw four antibiotic pills into her mouth and crumpled to the floor with her eyes closed.

The normal dose was two pills. She could have taken two pounds of antibiotics and lived to tell the tale. The nurse chortled, recovered, and tried to act like her laugh was a cough.

I saw her in a patient room and asked, "You're feeling suicidal?"

"Yes, I want to die! If this doesn't kill me, I'll do something else!"

"Fortunately, amoxicillin is not going to kill you. Since you're feeling suicidal…"

Her cell phone rang; she interrupted to answer. Her voice quaking, she said, "Hello, Kyle. I'm in the ER; I tried to kill myself."

She cradled the phone and scowled. I watched her for what seemed an eternity.

She wiped her tears, smiled blissfully, and said, "Oh, sweetheart, I love you so much! I'm so happy!"

I excused myself. The next patient was an attractive young woman in her twenties. She had lower abdominal pain.

I asked about her past medical history and her current problem. I asked about her last menstrual period.

She said, "I'm TS. I don't have menstrual periods."

"Oh, okay. TS. Well, we will need to do some blood tests and check a urine sample. We'll need to do a pelvic exam."

"Sure, if you say so."

I left the room. TS? What is that? A rare syndrome? I probably should know.

I pulled out a textbook and looked up TS; I couldn't find anything.

A few minutes later I asked the nurse to ready the patient for a pelvic exam. I walked in the room and her legs were up in the stirrups.

I said, "One thing I should've clarified earlier, what is TS? Is that a hormonal problem?"

"Trans-sexual."

The term settled in like humidity.

I stammered, "So you're a trans-sexual?"

"Yes."

This was suddenly awkward with a capital AWK. I tried to figure out what to ask next.

"So, uhh, well, are you a man or a woman?" What a weird question.

"I'm undergoing gender reassignment. I'm a preoperative female." What does that mean? Preoperative female? I was in deep water.

"So are you—do you currently have—a penis or a vagina?" Weirder question.

"I still have my penis. I'm scheduled for gender reassignment surgery in a few months. I'm currently on hormone therapy."

"I guess we don't need to do a pelvic exam." I fled from the room in a state of discombobulation.

⊞　⊞　⊞

I heard a commotion in the ER. I looked up from my chart as a naked, morbidly obese woman trotted past—out for a little jog. Her blubbery body jiggled like a jello salad mold knocked off the dinner table.

I stepped out in the hall as she ran down the corridor. She held out her hand and slapped the glass doors on several patient rooms as she lumbered by. The security guards chased and grabbed her by each arm. She did not try to fight.

She hollered, "Woo hoo! Check it out baby! Woo hoo!" She shook her hips back and forth and tossed her head side to side. They attempted to wrap a blanket around her, but she fought the efforts to cover her up.

They began walking her back to her room buck-naked. She stopped walking and sang something unintelligible. Then she obediently walked back to her room—a Lady Godiva of sorts. The psychiatric patient was well known for attention-seeking stunts.

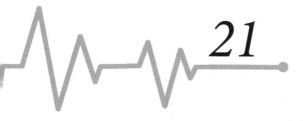

21

I was offered a job in Portland at Brookwood Hospital—a good fit since the emergency medicine residents rotate there. I was pleased to have the opportunity to teach. I was familiar with the doctors in the group because I rotated there. I was content. The light at the end of the tunnel was very close.

Missy and I were excited about starting a new chapter. We anticipated having time on our hands to recreate and relax. Our journey had been filled with delayed gratification and we were ready to reap the benefits. We were no longer in the vortex of academia, spinning around the axis of a diploma. Now, we could set our goals with much more freedom. Finally, we'd have time for each other. We were both ready to dive into the next chapter of our life.

Noah took a job at a different hospital in Portland. He proposed to Suzie and they got married shortly after.

Our graduation party was a blast. We had a bonfire near Mount Hood and barked at the moon.

Noah was a bit snockered. He walked up with a silly grin, "I like that hat. Can I have it?"

I said, "No."

"Can I wear it?"

"I don't want your lice or scabies on my hat."

He snatched the baseball cap from my head and bolted. I gave chase a few steps into the dark, but he ran like a rabid bear was foaming at his heels. He ran around a building and circled back.

He looked like a total dork, sprinting with no one behind. Someone said, "He thinks you're still chasing him!" We laughed as he zoomed past.

He ran full-throttle into a tangle of blackberry thorns about waist high. He was three feet deep before he realized his error. He stood in tortured limbo and then forced himself out. He was wearing shorts; his legs looked like he had been whipped. He moaned, cussed, and chuckled. I laughed until tears ran down my cheeks.

I felt very close to my fellow residents even though I met them just three years earlier. The pressure cooker of residency created strong bonds—lifetime bonds. We were nervous about being on our own, but the enthusiasm of finally being done with training lit the evening with excitement.

The light at the end of the tunnel was moving. The light was moving toward us, at a rapid speed.

Noah and I were oblivious to the locomotive about to strike us head-on and drag us down the tracks.

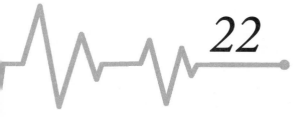

22

I worked at Brookwood for six months during residency and the atmosphere was friendly and cooperative, a bit less edgy than the University. Brookwood treats a suburban crowd: more heart attacks, less stabbings, more stable families with sick children, less homeless drug users. At any ER, the poor, the weak, and the homeless make up a disproportionate percent of patients compared to the surrounding population.

Brookwood is in a nice area, but approximately one third of our patients are not insured. At the University, it's more like three fourths. One reason is the poor have nowhere else to go; the ER is their safety net. Another is that sub-par behavioral choices, such as playing with power tools while drunk, are more common with people who can't gain or hold employment. An alcoholic has a hard time keeping a job, and they end up in the ER more than the average person.

Brookwood was able to attract good doctors and nurses, making it a pleasant place to work. My transition was seamless; my first two months had gone without a bump. I saw an average number of patients per shift: about twenty in eight hours. I didn't have any patient complaints, missed diagnoses, or negative interactions.

Missy and I enjoyed our new freedom and the time on our hands. We camped, biked, and traveled. We reconnected with family and friends. I felt like we were settling in to our new life; I liked it.

⊡ ⊡ ⊡

I was working a night shift. I'm often foggy during night shifts, but I felt sharp and buoyant. Night shifts are a hazard. Shift workers have as much cardiac risk as someone who smokes a pack of cigarettes a day. The people who are up at night are a different breed; the freaks come out at night.

I picked up the next chart—rectal pain, possibly a hemorrhoid on an abscess. The patient was a middle-aged rotund man who looked like a Basset Hound. His jowls quivered as he spoke, "Doc, I was in the shower and I slipped and fell. I felt a little pain in my rear, but I didn't think much of it. I started looking around for my shaving cream can and couldn't find it." He stopped talking and looked at me.

I said, "What happened? Does your tailbone still hurt? What about the shaving cream can?" I had a sinking feeling.

He said, "Well, I was wondering if maybe the can got lodged in my rear somehow. It's unusual, but I almost feel like something's stuck where the sun don't shine."

I was happy to play along with the charade; it was easier for both of us. I said, "OK. I guess we need to find out. I'll order an X-ray."

The X-ray showed a full sized shaving cream can in his rectum. He must have had some practice to get to that level.

The general surgeon was not very excited about getting a call from me at 2 a.m. He had a few choice words to describe the situation. The patient was taken to the operating room and the can was removed under general anesthesia.

The glamour of emergency medicine: puke, stool, and rectal shaving cream cans.

My next patient said, "Doc, can you keep a secret? I need some help bad, man!"

"I can keep a secret. What's bothering you?"

"You sure you can keep a secret? This is very important info."

"Go ahead."

He looked around suspiciously. He walked over to the sink and began inspecting it. He looked under the sink. I asked, "What are you looking for?"

"Bugs."

"There are no bugs. The rooms are cleaned after each patient."

"Not insects, bugs."

"Oh, listening devices?" I was pretty sure what his problem was.

He nodded his head slowly and placed his finger to his mouth in a silent hush signal.

"I'm sure this room is not electronically bugged."

He spoke in a hushed tone, "I've figured out a plot. Man, this is big, very big. I've written it all down. Tom Brokaw is Satanic. He made a deal with Satan to give him fame and fortune. He's watching us through our television sets. Brokaw, Bin Ladin, and Brittney Spears are using radiation from the television set to turn everyone into mindless jihadists—like terrorists, Muslim terrorists. The Angel Gabriel spoke to me and warned of the plot. I have to get this information into the hands of Billy Graham and the FBI. Can you help? I have it all written in this notebook."

As soon as he told me he had figured out a plot, I knew his illness.

He handed me a notebook with a magic marker title: The Book of Life, which was chock full of handwritten diagrams and illegible flow charts. I reviewed his chart and read he had schizophrenia. He needed to be admitted and his meds adjusted.

We see mentally ill patients almost every shift. Schizophrenia is a thought disorder with measurable biochemical anomalies in the brain. Being mentally ill carries a stigma, but schizophrenia is as real and biological as diabetes or cancer. The general public often confuses schizophrenia with multiple personality disorder, which is a different illness.

MIRACLES and MAYHEM in the ER

Multiple personality disorder (MPD) is an emotional disorder, as opposed to a thought disorder like schizophrenia. A patient with MPD will display multiple distinct identities and personalities. MPD is a psychological defense mechanism that patients will use to isolate trauma in their lives, often childhood sexual abuse. "That happened to Sue. I'm Barbara."

There are multiple subtypes of schizophrenia. Paranoid schizophrenics imagine gonzo plots and sinister scenarios, like this patient. Catatonic schizophrenics withdraw completely, often holding bizarre postures for hours on end. The hallmark of disorganized schizophrenia is a complete scrambling of thought processes. These patients will say things like, "Why do you look at me so smiling as the rabbit crawled, red and blue?"

Schizophrenia is caused by faulty dopamine activity in the brain. Patients with schizophrenia are prone to homelessness and drug abuse. They may self-medicate with illegal drugs; they also share the cruel streets with drug addicts and alcoholics. Bad habits are contagious.

After seeing the schizophrenic patient, I was about to sew up the scalp of an elderly woman who had tripped while getting up to go to the restroom. I saw a policeman bring in a handcuffed young man covered in bloody dirt.

The policeman removed the cuffs and left the patient in the room. A nurse gave the man a gown and pulled the curtain so he could change in privacy.

Max was the other emergency doc on that night. The policeman told him, "This is Jimmy, a bad drunk if there ever was one. Get this: we got a call about a domestic disturbance in a middle class neighborhood. Neighbors were concerned about yelling. I thought I'd tell them to quiet down and that'd be the end of it.

"I walked up to the quiet house. I knocked on the front door and it flew open. Jimmy burst out the door, wild eyed and sweaty. He almost knocked me over. He must've seen me coming and was waiting at the door; he opened it the second I knocked. He sloppily ran to his car in the driveway, cranked it, and squealed into the road.

"I radioed for backup. He took off down the neighborhood street doing about fifty. As he hit the first turn, he lost control and left the road, flipping the car upside down. The car ended up in a neighbor's front yard. I pulled my pistol and ran down; he was squished upside down on the ceiling of the car, dazed and mumbling. I called off the backup since he's just an out-of-control drunk half-wit. You got to be a pretty poor driver to roll your car within one hundred yards of your house.

"He's banged up so I brought him here. He has a few cuts on his head and arm and some glass in his hair. I didn't see any serious injuries.

"I spoke with his wife; she said he gets out of control when he drinks. She wasn't injured."

Max said, "Sounds like a rip-roaring time. I will check him out after the nurse gets him tucked in. Thanks."

I went back to the laceration repair. I had just finished when I heard a loud commotion. A nurse stuck her head in the room and said, "You need to check this out." I apologized to the patient and walked out, curious.

The nurse said, "I went in to check on that patient and he wasn't in the room. I walked out and told the policeman he was gone. He said it was impossible since he had been standing right outside the room the entire time. We both went back in and I looked up and saw a ceiling panel out of place. That guy is running around up in the crawl space!"

The policeman was looking up at the hole in the ceiling and talking on his radio. About the same time we heard a crashing from a room next door. Jimmy began yelling, "Ha-HA!" over and over. He stomped on the ceiling, knocking down fiberglass panels.

In the next room over, he stamped the light fixture. Fluorescent shards rained down on an elderly patient. She seemed confused to have glass suddenly sprayed over her. When the nurse hurried her out, she said, "Sorry to be a bother." Her silver hair glittered with glass.

More pieces of ceiling panels fell. The panels separated from the water sprinkler heads, and the sprinklers hung solo.

A tattooed man and his girlfriend ran out of the next room. He was looking at the ceiling with his arm across his face, "Something heavy is crashing around up there!"

A nurse wheeled a morbidly obese woman into the hall and the patient hyperventilated. "I need my inhalers!"

Debris rained down on the schizophrenic patient; he looked terrified as he was escorted out. Who knows what he thought about it all. I'm sure he wrote a new chapter in The Book of Life.

Jimmy screamed, "Pig, come get me!" He sent more and more crashing glass and fiberglass down. Officer Sampson pulled his gun and looked quite freaked.

I also was freaked, as was Max and the rest of the staff. Freaked all around.

The nursing staff moved patients out of that section of the ER.

Jimmy's foot plunged through the ceiling. The officer aimed his gun at the Adidas; I saw his grip tighten. I thought he was going to shoot Jimmy's foot. I could imagine him shooting the foot, splattering toes and rubber against the wall. I was relieved when Jimmy pulled his foot back.

He scurried around like a mouse in a cheap apartment; we weren't sure where he was, or how far he could roam in the space.

He yelled, "Come get me, squeally cop!" and, "You ain't so in control now, are you, boy?"

Officer Sampson trained his gun on the ceiling the entire time, shifting around quickly like he was in a shootout.

Max, one of my best buddies, and I watched the drama.

Jimmy had knocked down so many ceiling panels that he and Officer Sampson made eye contact. He straddled an open space standing on ceiling joists. Jimmy held a metal bar and said, "I'm going to beat you like I shoulda beat Carla."

Officer Sampson had his gun zeroed on Jimmy; he said, "You have five seconds to put down the bar before I open fire."

Max and I looked at each other with widened eyes. He said, "I really hope he doesn't smoke him, or our night is about to get really ugly."

I could visualize it: Bang, bang. Blood spurting. He clutches his chest. His body slowly tips forward and falls through the hole, landing with a sickening thud. People scream and run. Placing him on a gurney. More screams.

Death rattle breathing.

"Please, Doc, don't let me die."

Intubation. Blood flying everywhere. Placing chest tubes. Opening his chest and holding his tattered heart.

A police officer forever scarred; a life wasted due to unspeakable stupidity.

Luckily, Jimmy ran laterally into a different space, and we could no longer see him. Officer Sampson looked like he would probably rather be at Krispy Kreme.

Officer Sampson's backup finally arrived, probably fifteen officers. They flooded in like commandos in a hostage situation. They had unusual equipment: night vision goggles, automatic weapons, and ropes. They only lacked a grenade launcher.

Jimmy looked down on the platoon of cops; he seemed to be enjoying himself. He flipped birds, yelled insults, and grabbed his crotch.

The police moved a ladder into the room. One said, "Sir, come down the ladder or we will taser you." He pointed the hand held taser at Jimmy, who was standing above the policemen, in full view.

A taser is an electroshock weapon that causes involuntary muscle contraction and pain. The policeman had a type of taser that fires dart-like electrodes connected to the unit by wires. The darts go through clothes and into skin. A strong electrical charge courses through the wires and causes severe pain and incapacitation. The taser causes muscle and sensory nerves to fire, and is not dependent on pain to incapacitate people. The electrodes have barbs like fishhooks; we often have to work them out of a patient's skin.

Jimmy was bobbing and weaving like a kid playing dodge ball, "Hey, Luke Skywalker! You can stick that laser gun up yours!" The police officer said nothing, and kept the taser zeroed on Jimmy.

Jimmy stood for about five seconds in silence; his head moving back and forth with his hands out front, a cocky smirk on his face, his eyebrows jumping up and down. The policeman calmly fired the taser; it struck him in the middle of his chest.

Bulls-eye.

Jimmy fell to the floor screaming. His muscles spasmed; he herked and jerked on the ground.

Pause.

"O.K., Jimmy, climb down the ladder."

"Pigs!"

Just like the Price Is Right, there was a buzzing sound. Wrong answer.

He screamed. His body contracted in a rictus of misery.

I wondered if his hair would catch fire: an electrocution.

Jimmy lay silent.

He moaned softly. He said, "O.K., O.K.,! I'm coming down!" He stood and slowly backed down the ladder.

When his feet were within reach, they attacked like a defensive line released on a lone quarterback. They slammed him to the floor, handcuffed his hands behind his back, and snapped shackles on his feet.

Jimmy was placed in a secure room, handcuffed to a stretcher. Max ordered an intramuscular shot of a tranquilizer. Jimmy became much more sedate.

Max did a complete physical exam. He X-rayed his neck, chest, and right arm. He CT scanned his brain. All of these tests were normal. They obtained a drug screen that was only positive for alcohol, no other drugs.

I thought to myself about how destructive abusing alcohol can be. Of course, using alcohol responsibly never hurt anyone, but it costs society more than all of the street drugs combined. Normal usage of alcohol is healthier than teetotalism, but abuse carries a heavy penalty. It causes people to behave quite stupidly, as evidenced by Jimmy. With repeated abuse, it destroys the brain, liver, and digestive system. It ruins families and causes accidents. On the scale of personal destruction, it is right in the middle compared to other drugs of abuse—less destructive than heroin, crack, or methamphetamines, but much more so than marijuana, LSD, and mushrooms. It is about like powder cocaine.

Max spent thirty minutes stitching up his lacerations on his arm, leg, and face, and removing the taser darts. Jimmy was much more cooperative.

He said, "Doc, what have I done? I've never been arrested before. I have always had a job. I'm taking classes to become a commercial airline pilot. I can just be such an idiot when I get drunk. I've lost many friends due to drinking. I've got to quit drinking."

The cops cuffed him and led him to jail.

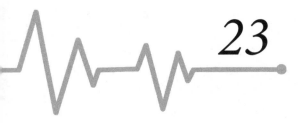

23

Noah and I loaded the mountain bikes. We were covered in mud; Missy and Suzie looked like female mud wrestlers. We drove toward Portland.

I said, "Listen to this! A drunk guy climbed up into the crawl space of the ER and destroyed the ceiling in several rooms. He taunted the cops and got tasered. Twice!" I told the whole story and said, "That's a pretty big penalty for a bender. The damage to the ER was over fifty grand. I'm sure he got jail time and a felony record."

Suzie said, "Some people can't drink. My friend quit drinking because he'd always do stupid things. The last straw was waking up in the morning, naked on the neighbor's couch, with the neighbors standing over him."

I said, "That was the freakiest shift I've had since graduation. It's weird, not having an attending to rely on or ask questions. How do you feel, being on your own?"

Noah said, "It's nerve wracking. I lie awake after shifts wondering if I should've done this or that."

"Yeah, me too. I hope to go for a while with no big mistakes, to gain confidence."

"I'm afraid I've lost confidence recently. I had an excruciating patient last week. I'm going to get a bleeding ulcer from this one." Noah told the story of a patient that would change both our lives.

⊞   ⊞   ⊞

Noah was at work when he heard the paramedic radio. Over the wailing siren, the paramedic yelled, "We're bringing a critically ill 50-year-old with crushing chest pain. His EKG looks like he's having a heart attack. The patient requested to go to Brookwood, but we're coming there since you're closer!"

A few minutes later the patient arrived, his sallow skin glistening with sweat. He clutched his left hand to his chest—the universal sign for a heart attack. His wife and adult son rushed in.

Noah said, "When did your chest pain start?"

"I thought I was having indigestion all day today, but it got much worse about fifteen minutes ago. It feels like an elephant's sitting on my chest."

"Have you had heart problems?"

"No. I've always been healthy. I've had more heartburn this week. I've noticed the discomfort is worse when I walk up the stairs. I had a hard time playing golf yesterday due to the discomfort."

"Are you short of breath?"

No answer. Noah looked at him; his eyes were open, but vacant. The nurse shouted, "He's in V tach!"

Noah glanced at the cardiac monitor; his heart rhythm had deteriorated into chaotic vibrations. Mr. Bristol lost consciousness.

Noah spun and grasped the defibrillation paddles. "Charge to two hundred joules!"

He slammed them to his chest. "All clear?"

Shock.

His chest heaved like he had been punched in the back. His wife cried out and turned her face into her son's chest; he put both arms around her.

The heart jump-started and cranked back up. Mr. Bristol hurtled back to earth from the heavens and landed with a thud; a primal groan escaped from his lips.

Mr. Bristol glanced about, his lips agape, "What happened?"

The smell of charred flesh and burnt chest hair snaked around the room.

"Your heart stopped. We shocked you back into a normal heart rhythm. I think you're having a heart attack."

"A heart attack? My heart stopped?"

The tech ripped the EKG off the printer, and handed it to Noah. The EKG showed the rounded elevation of the EKG baseline signaling a heart attack—tombstones.

Noah said, "You're having a heart attack. I'll call the cardiologist and they'll take you to the cath lab. They will attempt to open the blocked blood vessel to prevent your heart from permanent damage. They'll thread a catheter into your heart to open the blockage. That's called angioplasty."

Noah ordered several meds—blood thinners and rhythm stabilizers.

A few minutes later, the cardiologist called back, "I'm in the cath lab right now with a tough case. I won't be done in less than an hour. We don't have a backup team. You should transfer this patient to another hospital. I've alerted my partner, Dr. Heller, who's on his way to the ER to help you manage the patient and help with the transfer."

Noah hung up. Mr. Bristol's heart was dying, and the longer it took to open up the vessel in his heart, the more permanent damage. Every minute passed was heart muscle scorched. The gold standard for treatment is to cath the patient within thirty minutes of arriving at the hospital.

Noah returned to Mr. Bristol's room. "I spoke with our cardiologist on call. He's in the middle of another emergency heart procedure. We need to transfer you to another hospital. I'm working on it."

"O.K., whatever you say; I just want to get better. I wish they would've listened to me and taken me to Brookwood. My doctor works there." His wife and son both scowled slightly.

Noah replied, "The paramedics have a protocol to bring unstable patients to the nearest hospital; a critically ill patient is better served in an ER than an ambulance."

Dr. Heller showed up a few minutes later. He went to manage Mr. Bristol while Noah worked on the transfer.

Noah took a call from a cardiologist at the nearest hospital. "We can't take him now. We have a patient in our ER that needs our cath lab."

Noah hung up in disbelief. The chance of having two heart attack patients simultaneously was vanishingly rare. That is why there was only one team on call. A team is composed of a cardiologist, two nurses, and a tech; ready twenty-four hours a day, three hundred and sixty five days a year. To have two teams on call would be wasteful.

Except for the once-a-year patient—Mr. Bristol.

Noah told the secretary, "Call every hospital in the area. We have to get him out of here as fast as possible. Get an ambulance team here now."

The clock showed that Mr. Bristol had been in the ER for thirty-seven minutes: far too long. Noah felt a gnawing in his gut; the stress chewed.

Dr. Heller walked out of Mr. Bristol's room. Noah explained the problems with the transfer and asked, "What do you think about giving him a clot buster? Then he wouldn't need to go to the cath lab?"

The cardiologist replied, "That's an option, but if I were the patient, I'd rather wait for the cath lab rather than risk the devastating complications of clot busting medicine."

Noah said, "I'll get another EKG and see if it's changed."

While the tech was doing the second EKG, Noah told Mr. Bristol about the discussion, "A clot buster is a medicine we put in your IV that dissolves all clots in the body. It will often abort a heart attack and used to be the standard treatment for heart attacks. We've discovered catheterization works better and is safer. A clot buster medicine, or CB, has a fairly high incidence of bleeding complications, including bleeding into the brain—causing severe brain damage, or bleeding to death."

Noah took the second EKG to Dr. Heller. "Look at this one; it looks much better."

He said, "True. I feel better about the decision to transfer rather than give a clot buster. His EKG no longer meets criteria for CB treatment. Now, it's clearly better to transfer to a different hospital, even with the delay."

A cardiologist from a third hospital called, "We can take your patient. We'll be ready as soon as he gets here. The team's already been mobilized."

Fifty-nine minutes. He still had to be transported to the cath lab at the other hospital—so much for the thirty-minute window. Noah felt nauseated.

Noah explained the situation to the family; the nurses prepared for transport. The paramedics hustled him out with the family jogging behind the stretcher. The paramedics fired up the sirens and then the sound drained away.

One hour, twelve minutes.

⊞　⊞　⊞

Missy said, "That poor man! What happened?"

Suzie said, "I'd be so angry if I was his family. Why didn't they take him to Brookwood?"

Noah said, "I don't know what happened, but I'm sure his heart was permanently damaged. They couldn't take him to Brookwood; their protocol says to take unstable patients to the nearest hospital."

I said, "It doesn't sound like you could've done anything differently or better than you did." I wanted to dissect it and talk about the choices, but I tried to act like it wasn't a big deal. Noah needed support, not an inquiry.

He said, "I've been over the case multiple times in my mind. I think I did everything I could do, but I feel terrible."

I felt empty. All of our training and preparation for treating patients, and this is how it turned out—a completely fried heart in a treatable patient. I did not want to belabor the point with Noah, but this was a worst-case scenario. All our anxieties about being on our own, and a patient being injured on our watch had been realized. Noah did not do anything wrong, but this man was injured due to unfortunate circumstances. I thought about Cannibal Cullison, whose heart was so damaged he couldn't walk across the room without panting. Mr. Bristol was probably going to be crippled, badly.

I suspected Mr. Bristol and his ruined heart would be a frequent visitor to Noah's thoughts, and nightmares.

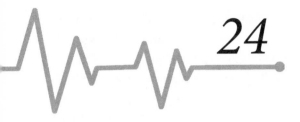

My alarm went off at 5 a.m. I clamored out of bed and splashed water on my face. I try to get eight hours of sleep, but—following my pre-night shift routine—I had set my alarm for five hours of sleep. The more I sleep the afternoon before a night shift, the better I will feel at 4 a.m.

I drove out to the Gorge and windsurfed until my hands ached and my entire body was fatigued. I ran a few errands. At 4 p.m., I took a hot shower, ate a big meal, and lay down with a book. I turned on my white noise maker and pulled the blackout window blinds.

I planned to sleep from 5 p.m. to 10 p.m. and then go to work at 11 p.m., well rested and ready for battle. At six, I was still wide-awake, so I took an over-the-counter sleep aid. The OTC sleep aids are antihistamines, like Benadryl. At eight, I took another.

I lay in bed, worried. Nine p.m.

I was going to feel horrible if I showed up at work and had not slept at all. I felt fuzzy headed from the Benadryl but not sleepy. I was getting anxious, but I tried to relax. Think happy thoughts.

What if a dying baby came in, or a complicated sick person? I needed to be firing on all cylinders. There was no attending I could rely on if I couldn't think straight. At ten, my alarm went off, and I had not slept at all.

I was stressed and exhausted. I had purposely gotten less than optimal sleep, an active day with vigorous exercise, and three sleeping pills. I shaved, dressed, and crawled into my car. My eyelids were heavy as I drove to work. I rolled down the window hoping the cool night air would wake me.

I walked into the brightly-lit ER with a cup of coffee. The lights annoyed me. I felt a mix of nausea, exhaustion, irritability, and doom. I felt like a swath of pink itchy fiberglass insulation was wrapped around me, separating me from others. I wondered if I looked as horrible as I felt.

I looked at the chart rack; there were five patients waiting to be seen. The waiting room was full. It would be hours before I could see the patients already waiting. I was going to be running hard all night—running until my feet ached and lungs burned. I dreaded what I would feel like in the early a.m.

I went to see the first patient. As I was taking the history, I forgetfully repeated questions.

A few hours later, I was fully mired. Nurses were asking me when I was going to send so-and-so home, what was the plan for room nine, room twelve was anxious to leave. I looked at the chart rack and there were seven charts waiting to be seen. I was treading water with my chin barely above the surface.

I longed to find an empty room and lie down. Sleep sounded incredibly inviting. I blinked for several seconds; each blink was a temptation to leave my eyes closed.

One in five first-year residents admits to a fatigue-induced mistake that injured a patient, one in twenty to a fatal mistake—a death.

My thoughts of a soft pillow were interrupted by the paramedic radio, "We have a 17-year-old with chest pain. He's in shock; his blood pressure is 70 systolic. He doesn't look good. We'll be there in ten."

I wanted to say, "Don't bring him here. Take him somewhere else. Anywhere else. For his own good. Please!"

As we waited, I brushed away the cobwebs and thought about the possibilities. I was surprised by his age. We see older people with heart attacks, but not 17-year-olds.

The paramedics wheeled in a tall, handsome, black teenager clutching his chest. The paramedic reported, "Myron awoke with crushing chest pain. He says he can't breathe; his oxygen level is low. He feels like something is squeezing his chest.

"When did the pain start?"

He pulled his oxygen mask to the side to speak, "I was asleep. Bam! A strong pain hit me right in the chest. I thought I was shot or something." He stopped talking and labored to breathe, "I can't hardly breathe."

Watching him struggle, my exhaustion was momentarily overcome by the clear peril of the situation. I knew something was seriously wrong. His blood pressure and oxygen levels were very low and he looked like he could go into cardiac arrest at any moment. He was barely hanging on.

He was seventeen.

He was in shock. In common vernacular, shock means stunned. In medicine, shock means low blood pressure. Cardiogenic shock occurs when the heart is not beating strongly enough to maintain a blood pressure. Hypovolemic shock is caused by low blood volume, usually from bleeding or dehydration. Septic shock occurs when overwhelming infection causes everything to malfunction.

His heart was racing. He did not have a fever. I listened to his heart and lungs—normal. I said, "Get two large IVs and run two liters of fluid wide open. Let's get an EKG, a stat chest X-ray, and cardiac labs."

166

His parents and girlfriend rushed in. Myron's father introduced himself; he had a fatherly charisma. He immediately reminded me of my buddy Fred's dad; they had similar mannerisms. His face radiated warmth, even in the midst of an emergency.

Myron's girlfriend looked like a young Whitney Houston. Myron was a high school basketball star, being recruited by several universities, and his father was a pastor, just like Fred's.

His father asked, "Doctor, what's wrong with him?"

"I don't know yet."

I ran through the possibilities in my fatigued mind. I said, "Myron, a blood clot to your lungs could cause these symptoms. Blood clots usually form in people who have cancer, a blood clotting disorder, or recent surgery."

"I don't have any of that." He gripped his chest and sweat dripped from his chin. "My chest feels like somebody's standing on it. I can't get air!" His father looked quizzical and his mother alarmed.

Another possibility was a pneumothorax—leaking air from a lung. Sometimes a lung will spontaneously leak. Air expelled rapidly can cause a tension pneumothorax. The heart and lungs are crushed in the chest cavity by the high air pressure—not compatible with life. When this diagnosis is made, a needle is quickly stabbed into the chest to relieve the tension. A chest tube is placed afterward. I doubted Myron had a pneumothorax because that is usually diagnosed by a lack of breath sound on one side, and his lung exam was normal.

A heart attack seemed unlikely in a 17-year-old, unless he used coke or meth. The basketball star Len Bias died of a heart attack due to cocaine. I hated asking about drugs in front of his family, but time was of the essence.

"Do you use illegal drugs?

He replied, "No, I don't do that stuff." I ordered a urine drug screen to verify.

An aortic dissection, due to weakness in the aortic wall, was possible. Blood flows into the wall of the aorta instead of through it, like a faulty water hose that develops a second passage. The flow of blood is reduced and blood pressure drops, just as the hose's water pressure would drop and the flow would become chaotic.

My brother's college roommate dropped dead from an aortic dissection due to Marfan's syndrome. Marfan's, a connective tissue disorder, is a common cause of premature death due to aortic dissection. Marfan's patients are usually tall and lanky, like Myron. Abe Lincoln probably had Marfan's, a fairly common disease.

Another possibility was pericardial tamponade. The pericardium is a fibrous sack surrounding the heart. If fluid builds up in that space, the pressure will crush the heart. This causes cardiogenic shock. Fluid can develop due to trauma, infection, kidney disease, or cancer. In the ER, the pressure can be temporarily relieved, by sticking a needle into the sack. The permanent solution is surgically opening a hole in the sack.

Myron could have a viral infection of his heart–viral myocarditis– that would cause his heart to beat like a flat basketball, also causing cardiogenic shock.

He could have a clot or an infection on a heart valve causing an obstruction of blood flow, like a clogged pipe. The valves of the heart may develop clots, usually due to an infection called endocarditis. Endocarditis is most often seen with abnormal valves causing turbulent blood flow, or with IV drug abusers. Infections fly from the heart like a medieval archer launching an onslaught of flaming arrows. The blazing arrows cause fires wherever they land—in the brain, in the lungs, or wherever blood flows. The fiery infections cause the fever that accompanies endocarditis.

Many IV drug abusers with endocarditis are taken piece by piece until there is not much left to take, and they keep shooting blow and arrows. Myron might snort coke, but I doubted IV cocaine or heroin. The son of a preacher man looked like a healthy teenager, if he lived to see the following day.

Nevertheless, I had a lot to figure out and not much time. I willed my fatigue away. The fatigue would return, but hopefully it would stay away long enough.

Myron did not look well, his face a mix of pain and weakness. He whispered, "I think I'm going to die today."

His girlfriend said, "No you're not, baby! Hang in there, Myron! You're a fighter!" She fiercely wiped away tears.

His father said decisively, "We need to pray."

His girlfriend nodded.

The three of them joined hands in a corner of the room and prayed for Myron. They prayed in the soulful, energetic way I had seen at Fred's church. Myron's mother punctuated the reverend's words with "Yes, Jesus! We praise your name, Lord!"

I felt an odd sense of personal attachment to the family, even though I had just met them. They struck a powerful chord into my formative years and reminded me—not only of friends—but of the culture and forces that shaped me. They reminded me of home.

Myron's mother began to weep during her prayers. She said, "Lord, please save my baby!" I lost my ability to speak and averted my face lest anyone see my tears.

I was more focused than I had ever been; I needed to figure it out fast. Myron appeared not long for this world; he was glazed and sleepy. He was not old enough to journey to heaven.

Not on my watch.

I reviewed the chest X-ray and EKG. Both were normal, making a heart attack, viral heart infection, or pneumothorax less likely.

I had to decide if it was more likely a pulmonary embolus or an aortic dissection. They required different types of CT scans; both use a large amount of toxic CT dye. Two scans in one day greatly increased the risk of permanent kidney damage.

Most people in shock are easy to diagnose and treat. The septic person with pneumonia will have a cough and a fever. A heart attack is usually obvious on the first EKG, like the patient Noah treated. Myron was not easy to diagnose and therefore not easy to treat.

All of his organs were being damaged due to his prolonged low blood pressure—not enough oxygen was arriving to the organs and they were suffocating. I ordered dopamine to try to get his pressure out of the basement.

I rolled the dice and guessed an aortic dissection was more likely. He was tall and thin and had no risk factors for a pulmonary embolus.

I walked beside him to the CT scanner; I worried that he might crump and need intubation. I said, "Hang in there. We should have this figured out soon." His eyes seemed to search my face for clues about his fate. I tried to project confidence—confidence I did not have.

As I sat waiting on the scan, the darkness of the room and the hum of the scanner tempted me to put my head down. I would just rest for just a few seconds until the scan was done. I rested my head.

I slipped away.

Peace, warmth.

Quiet.

Stillness.

A nurse woke me, "Brent, the scan is done." I bolted upright. She looked at me, concerned.

A few minutes later, the radiologist called with the report—normal. At this point, there were a few possibilities. I did not have his urine drug screen results; it could be a drug-induced heart attack. He could have tamponade, although that would often be seen on CT scanning. A valve problem or a blood clot seemed most likely.

I returned to his room. His face was ashen, as much as a man with African blood can look pale. His father was also—ashes to ashes. Sweat drenched Myron's gown, and he breathed like he had sprinted a mile. He clutched as if there was something inside his chest murdering him: something violent, something deadly. I had to reap the Reaper, but I needed to find him first.

I racked my brain about what to do next. Fatigue closed in like dark walls. I sat. I stood. I walked. I gulped ice water. I sipped coffee.

I decided that I could get the most information, with the least risk, from a bedside cardiac ultrasound. That would show pericardial tamponade, viral infection, or valve problems. It wouldn't show a blood clot to the lung.

Myron was mumbling instead of talking. I wondered if I should intubate him. His blood pressure was still teetering on the precipice. He gasped and wheezed. He was in and out of consciousness. He looked like he might die at any moment and I still had no diagnosis. I said, "Let's prepare for intubation. He's worsening."

His father and mother dropped to their knees and began to pray, to plead with God to spare their son's life. Their hands were on each other's shoulders. His girlfriend hummed Amazing Grace as they prayed. Their desperation and love for their son was so raw and heartfelt that I nearly burst into tears—my emotions tattered due to fatigue.

The ultrasound tech arrived. The ultrasound of his heart showed normal valves, no signs of heart infection, but a dilated right ventricle. The right ventricle pumps blood into the lungs. It was stretched due to a downstream blockage. Something was blocking flow of blood out of the heart into the lungs: almost certainly a blood clot.

I ordered a blood thinner to treat the clot. There is significant danger to ordering blood thinner when the diagnosis is unclear. If he had blood in the sack around the heart, blood thinners would be catastrophic. I felt the diagnosis was all but certain, and I had ruled out bleeding. To delay longer could worsen his condition.

I ordered a VQ scan to confirm the diagnosis. VQ scan is not as accurate as a CAT scan, but I wanted to avoid another load of toxic dye. The scan showed a massive blood clot, almost completely blocking blood flow to his lungs. My relief was overwhelming to finally have a diagnosis. I felt like collapsing in fatigue.

I explained his diagnosis to his family. I said, "I believe he will be OK. We know what's wrong and we have good treatment for this."

His mother said, "Thank you, doctor. I believe God sent you to help my boy." Tears flowed freely down her cheeks.

My eyes stung, my chin trembled, and I just nodded. I couldn't speak. She squeezed my hand and smiled through her tears.

His labs returned normal. His drug screen was completely negative. I called the report to the ICU.

I finished my shift in an exhausted, nauseated haze. My thoughts barely made sense and I double-checked myself, but I escorted my remaining patients safely through the ER.

When the morning doctor arrived, there were six charts in the rack, and a full waiting room. He said, "Looks like you had a rough night." I smiled grimly. I still had hours of dictations before I could go home.

When I finally went home, I struggled on the drive and was asleep seconds after my head hit the pillow.

⊡　⊡　⊡

I called Fred that week. I told him how much his parents reminded me of Myron's. He joked, "You white folks think we're all alike."

He asked, "What happened to that guy? What caused that clot?"

I said, "I'm not sure. I'll check on him and let you know."

A few weeks later Fred called from his parent's house and he put his mom on the phone. She said, "We think about you often. Fred keeps us up to date. We're so proud of you. I know you'll be a fine doctor. God bless you, son. Come see us next time y'all are in Mississippi."

I missed home.

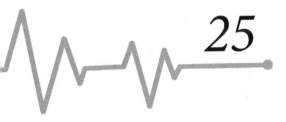

I thought about Myron's family and his near death experience for several days. I thought about religion, death, and race. Dealing with death, we have to be ready for the rituals and expectations regarding the afterlife. Most people believe they will live on after death—the body is a vehicle, transporting the soul. The majority of Americans believe in heaven, but some believe in reincarnation, eternal consciousness, or being reabsorbed into the life force. It is a rare person who believes we cease to exist when we die.

I often witness intimate spiritual moments due to the life and death nature of my work. As a physician, we have to walk a fine line. Most doctors try to separate themselves from the spiritual, leaving that to the patient, the family, and their chosen spiritual guides.

The patient's beliefs need to be respected, and the physician's beliefs can be part of the baggage. The prayers of the Jehovah's Witnesses did not viscerally move me, as I do not know any. The prayers of Myron's family were familiar and gripping. Their desperate pleas were haunting.

Our hospital is Catholic and prayers are broadcast daily. Once, a resident told me, "I'm an atheist and those prayers offend me." I thought, "You might be better off working elsewhere. Don't take a job at the Vatican if a crucifix gives you hives."

I think of faith as human nature on steroids. A belief in the divine often makes us better than we are, and many people of faith perform acts of unbelievable kindness and self-sacrifice.

At the other end, supernatural beliefs can lead to hate, murder, and destruction.

Religion has brought us many wars, but for many—peace.

Race has always interested me. We humans are tribal; we sort ourselves into groups—faith, race, and nationality are common tribes. There is nothing wrong with this per se, but this is a source of conflict around the world—me and my kind, us versus them. Racial and religious anger are potent, and often destructive, emotions.

The African American culture, while far from monolithic, is different than the white majority culture in many ways. Most eat, dress, recreate, speak, and worship differently. Our differences can be celebrated as opposed to being denied or being a source of prejudice and distrust.

Oregon is one of the whitest states in the Union and I see African American patients rarely; my schools in Mississippi were majority black. Many blacks on the West Coast have similar diction to the blacks in the South; whites on the West Coast do not sound like Southern whites. Myron's family brought back fond memories.

As a child we lived in the Smoky Mountains, on Signal Mountain, Tennessee. Isolated Appalachian hill people populated half of the mountain and the other half, where we lived, was a suburb of Chattanooga. Some of the rural folks did not welcome blacks and our mountain was all white. My mother did not like the segregation, as she embraced all people. Every week, we drove off the mountain to a housing project in Chattanooga where she would tutor children. My siblings and I would be the only white kids for miles, and spent the days running and playing with friends from the other side of the divide.

I remember sitting on my grandfather's porch in Mississippi after working on the farm: loading hay, or moving cattle. Most of the workers were black; we'd sit and drink iced tea in the late afternoon.

They would start ribbing each other or telling funny stories. One would make a comment and they would slap their knees and erupt in rib bursting laughter, then another would respond and they would double over. One might grasp another by the shoulder and shake gently, or slap each other on the back, as they continued their playful comments between gasps of contagious laughter. My grandfather laughed much more with them than with his white friends.

I grew up in an area known for racism and hostility between races, but there is also a rich tradition of friendship between people and cultures living side by side. That's what I prefer to remember.

Myron never had to be intubated and only spent a few days in the hospital. He had a previously undiagnosed clotting disorder and was placed on long-term blood thinners.

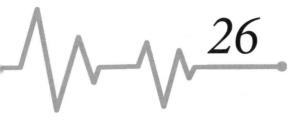

A few days later, Noah called, late in the evening. His demeanor was sullen and I knew something was wrong. He said, "I was leaving work tonight when a dude walked up to me in the parking lot and asked if I was Dr. Noah Jackson. I thought he might be a psycho freak I had seen as a patient.

"I didn't answer and I rotated away from him so he couldn't pin me down or get too near. I slid my hands out of my pockets and cautiously said, 'Why? Who are you?'

"He smiled—a creepy smile. I really thought he was a deranged weirdo. I continued to face him as I walked backwards toward the ER. My heart raced.

"The man said, 'I'm here to give you notice of a lawsuit.' He thrust an envelope at me.

"I snapped, 'Do you really think hiding in a dark parking lot is the best way to deliver a summons?' He turned and walked away."

My blood iced. The dreadful, dreaded lawsuit. A weirdo would have been better. That would be over and done with. A lawsuit will inflict pain for months, possibly years.

I said, "Who's suing you? That man who had a heart attack?"

"Yes. It was Mr. Bristol."

I did not know what to say next. It was sort of like him saying he had rectal cancer. I wanted to discuss how horrible and unfair it was, but he wanted to hear that everything was going to be all right. So I clumsily said nothing.

He continued, "The lawsuit is for economic damages, pain, and suffering caused by delayed treatment and mismanagement of a myocardial infarction."

I had to ask, "How much are they asking for?"

"Six million dollars. My malpractice insurance covers up to three million."

I swallowed hard.

◨　◨　◨

I changed into my scrubs in the dressing room. I told Nate, one of my partners, about Noah's lawsuit. He grimaced and said, "Noah's a great doctor, smart and thorough. If it can happen to him, it can happen to any of us. And I guess it will."

I said, "He's taking it pretty hard. He cares so much about his patients. He was upset the man was injured due to unfortunate circumstances. He's sad to be blamed, and he's worried about the professional and financial implications if he loses."

"It seems so unfair."

I noticed a deep abrasion on Nate's foot. I asked, "What happened?"

He looked sheepish. "I got into a bit of an altercation. Check out my hand." He held out his right hand and had scabs on the knuckles. Nate is a big guy who used to bike race; he lived with Lance Armstrong for a few years.

I smiled, "What happened?"

"A few months ago our car got broken into in front of our house. We live in a pretty nice area but there are some seedy characters that roam at night. Two days ago, I was in bed and I heard breaking glass.

"I jumped up and looked out the window; I saw someone sitting in the passenger seat of our car rifling through the glove compartment.

"I scrambled out the bedroom door in my underwear. My wife said, 'What are you doing?' I ran down the stairs: barefoot, no shirt on.

"I bolted onto the porch, jumped down the three front stairs. The man sprinted out of the car and ran across the street, and then continued to run down the sidewalk.

"I raced across the grass and hit the street at full speed.

"I took off running down the street. He looked back and saw me chasing him. He looked startled; he sped up."

I laughed, "That dude broke into the wrong car!"

He smiled, "The thought crossed my mind that it was a fairly idiotic thing to be doing; he could have a gun, a knife, or a friend down the street.

"But it was too late; I was enraged—on a mission. If he was going to knock out the window of my car, he was going to face the wrath.

"My killer instincts had kicked in."

I said, "The lion and the gazelle."

"I was gaining on him. He looked back again, I could see his eyes widen as he saw me closing the gap. I was silent: neither of us had said a word. He jumped off the sidewalk and tore though a dark yard, running between houses.

"I thought it was over. He had shoes on; it'd be impossible to keep up. I knew it was lunacy to continue; he could hide anywhere. I could've gotten all my teeth knocked out by a metal bar, or heard a gunshot—game over."

I smiled, "But you didn't stop?"

"Nope. I gave chase into the dark area between the houses. I felt my foot scrape something hard.

"I rounded the house and saw him run through hedges in the side of the yard. As I broke through the prickly bushes, I saw him much farther away, running through a front yard.

"I slowed; he was too far ahead.

"I saw him trip and fall. I heard a startled grunt. In a split second the sound went from startled to excruciating.

"He had dropped onto steps that led down to the street from a house. He dropped three feet, flipped onto his face, and collided with the concrete stairs. I was on him before he could stand.

"I sprung onto him with my legs straddling his chest and drew my fist back and landed about three punches to his nose and mouth. He yelled.

"My wife ran out and several neighbors showed up. There was palpable glee in the crowd: middle class yuppie revenge on the criminal. The organic latte sippers strike back!

"I was straddling the dude in my underwear. It was sprinkling. The cops showed up and cuffed him.

"There were about ten neighbors there. I felt ridiculous standing in my wet tighty-whities."

He said, "The officer asked me if I had any injuries. I showed him the scrapes on my foot and hand.

"He asked me if my hand was scraped for the same reason the dude's face was banged up.

"I said yes and he said, 'I think I will leave that out of the report.'"

I said, "That's hilarious! Doctor by day, crime fighter by night! Captain Underpants is here to save the day!"

▣ ▣ ▣

The shift crackled like dry firewood. I had seven patients in the ER and lots of balls in the air. I was talking on the phone to a long-winded admitting physician who was saying, "You know, I've spent a lot of time with this patient. She just will not do what I say. I get so sick of it, I mean, what am I supposed to do? She eats the wrong things, forgets to take her meds. I feel like pulling my hair out. She comes in to my office and asks the most irrelevant questions. A total nightmare, one time she asked me...." I was trying to figure out a way to end the conversation politely when I heard yelling. The nurses were attempting to restrain a patient.

I said, "John, I've got a situation here. I'm going to have to call you back." Click. I hung up without waiting to hear his response.

I quickly walked to the room with the combative patient. The patient was screeching a sing-song yodel that seemed more jubilant than angry. A policeman was standing outside the room.

The policeman said, "This is Tuan, he's a 22-year-old. I think he's Cambodian. He's high on something. He broke into his neighbor's apartment. They were asleep when they heard a noise in their living room. The man found Tuan standing on a chair, looking at the ceiling. The guy picked up a ceramic statue of the Virgin Mary and yelled for his wife to call the police.

"Tuan walked toward him, saying something about an evil lizard spirit. The man told him to stay away, but he walked toward him and made weird noises, clucking like a chicken and hissing. The man clocked him in the head with the statue of Mary and knocked him sideways. The wife threw glasses and beer bottles at him. I think they all missed or bounced off him. The man jumped on him and beat him in the face a few times. Tuan's about five feet tall and probably weighs a buck and a quarter.

"When I got there, the man was holding Tuan down; the man was pretty heavy. Tuan was making noises like an animal.

"We brought him here so you could check him out. After you finish, I'll take him down to the station and cite him for trespass, if he doesn't have any serious injuries."

I said, "O.K. Is he going to spend the night in jail?"

"I doubt it; he hasn't done anything violent. I am sure he's just fully loaded and wandered into that apartment. He was getting on my nerves driving over here; making his little weird noises and comments. I thought about stopping and tossing him off the bridge into the river, but I figured you good people would be more than happy to take care of him. His hand is cuffed to the stretcher."

When I entered, Tuan said—in a bizarre voice accompanied by an Asian accent— "Hello, sexy man boy." He had an eerie smirk on his face and wouldn't take his eyes off of me. I asked him what had happened and he said, "Fighting the forces of evil, sexy man boy." It did not seem that further questioning was likely to be helpful.

I examined him. His left eye was swollen shut. He had a laceration over his left ear. He had blood smeared around his swollen lips like smudged lipstick. I ordered CAT scans of his face and head to look for facial fractures or bleeding in his brain.

Thirty minutes later, I returned to Tuan's room. He was staring at a wall, then he turned his head slowly toward me. When he saw me, his eyes flamed like funeral pyres. He leapt over the bedrail in one smooth motion. I was astonished that a human could move so fast and with such catlike grace. He rushed toward me, burning.

My flight-or-fight reflex jolted. I jumped back into a corner, and braced for impact. I reflexively dropped my shoulder and threw my hands in front of my face.

He jerked violently sideways before he reached me. His arm was connected to the gurney by a metal handcuff and his forward motion was abruptly stopped with a painful clank.

He screamed in a guttural voice. He turned back toward me with a menacing leer. He began pulling the three hundred fifty pound bed rapidly across the floor. The wheel brakes were on—the bed skidded across the floor. He clawed at me.

I did not want him between the door and myself, so I made my move. As I rushed past, he gripped the back of my shirt with his free hand and yanked hard. My collar bit into my neck like a wire garrote.

I spun, struck his arm with my elbow, and broke free.

I bolted into the hall with him in pursuit. The bed crashed into the sliding glass door. He clamored into the hallway but his arm was anchored to the bed.

Several security guards, nurses, and techs surrounded him. He crashed the bed into the doors repeatedly. His eyes were fiercely on me; he ignored everyone else. He only wanted me.

I did not want to know why. I rubbed my neck.

He whipped his head side to side and bared his teeth, saliva dripping down his chin. His eyes bulged as if they were being pushed out from within. He stopped, raised his brow to the sky, and howled.

I said, "On three, we rush him. I will get his right leg. One. Two. Three." We charged and overpowered him. We lifted him back onto the gurney. He screamed and twisted. He arched his entire torso in the air, with feet and arms held down on the bed.

With two people on each appendage, we tied him to the gurney using soft restraints. He tried to pinch and scratch with his hands. I was holding an arm and he scratched me with his fingernails.

I said, "Give him the hammer." The hammer would put a silverback into a coma.

Tuan spit on Pablo, our nurse. Pablo gripped Tuan's nose, and twisted—hard. Tuan looked quite uncomfortable to have his nose suddenly sideways.

We placed a towel over his face and he growled. He yelled curses, nonsensical noises, and peculiar sexual requests.

The nurse rushed in with the tranquilizer and stabbed him in the thigh. He shook the towel off his face and said, "Thank you, your highness." He stuck out his tongue and made licking motions in the air. He said, "Evil lizard, evil lizard."

The policeman had been in a front office, writing his report. He showed up just as we had Tuan under control. He shook his head, "I guess Tuan bought himself a jail cell."

One of my partners, Dave, got on the overhead speaker and announced, "Paging Father Damien to room twelve. Father Damien to room twelve, please." He made the sign of the cross and said, "That guy needs an exorcism."

After about 15 minutes, the tranquilizers kicked in; he fell asleep. He had normal CT scans. The handcuffed wrist was pretty beat up with abrasions and several deep lacerations. I sewed up the lacerations on his wrist and face. His urine drug screen came back positive for methamphetamines.

Pablo walked up and said, "Como estas, sexy man boy?"

I asked, "What was that nose maneuver? Where did you learn that?"

He smiled and said in a soft voice, "That's the Guatemalan nose twist. Don't mess with me." He held up his hand and made a pinching motion, raised one brow, and pointed a finger at me. "I'm watching you, hombre."

With Tuan asleep, I continued on my shift. Instead of being shaken up, I felt invigorated, like I had just played a football game— Team A: the entire ER staff, Team B: Tuan. I was glad to be on the winning team. I felt charged and ready for the post-game dance.

I kept Tuan in the ER for about six hours; when he awoke, he was lucid and subdued. I told him what had happened. I talked with him about meth. I didn't moralize. I told him what I thought he should hear: meth is the meanest kid on the block and it itches to drive you to submission, to conquer you, to make a mistake out of you. It usually succeeds, like a parasite that kills its host.

He did not have much to say. He was probably in a short-circuited fog; a concoction of competing poisons and drugs. We released him into police custody.

I have seen many patients enslaved by meth. Meth is gruesomely seductive; one hit and the future addict is euphoric and energetic for days on end. They can work, do chores, and stay up all night dancing. Sleep an hour and do it all over again. Everything is better—food tastes better, music sounds better, every pleasure is magnified.

When the corresponding crash comes a few days later, just take a hit and start over again: never felt better. Most plan to use it once in a blue moon; they end up using it once in a blue sky. Some probably function higher than normal the first few months on meth.

After a while, they need meth just to feel normal. After days without sleep, they think and behave erratically. The euphoria gone, sadness and madness replace happiness and sanity. Like flesh eating worms, the sickness travels the body.

The worms crawl in and eat the flowers. The worms come to stay; they chew holes in coherence, ooze miserable slime, and lay their destructive eggs in every cranny. Many spend hours a day picking at their skin, digging for the worms that torment them. The scratches and scabs are the official uniform of the tweaker.

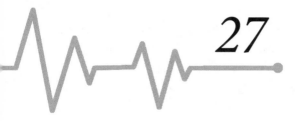

27

I arrived early for my shift and called the police to find out about Tuan. The police officer said, "He was calm in jail. But he didn't show up for his arraignment, so he has a warrant out for his arrest. I'm sure he is strung out somewhere. Those meth heads can't put it down."

I was a little surprised, but I guess I was naïve. I thought that maybe the combination of getting clobbered by a ceramic Virgin Queen of Heaven, sat on by a large man, arrested, cuffed, brought to the ER, restrained, becoming unrestrained, becoming unhinged, being restrained and-this-time-we-mean-it, getting cut, tranquilized, sewn, and lectured, and—finally—spending the night in jail could have convinced such a young guy to fly straight. But the sad reality is—most who get bitten, get eaten.

I did not tell Tuan anything that he didn't already know; he was already infected, infested. The worms were conquering another soul. Making a mistake out of Tuan.

I was assigned to the pediatric area of the ER. The ten brightly colored rooms are separate from the main ER so the young ones don't have to be exposed to bloody gore or to screaming Jimmy or Tuan.

The next patient was a 3-year-old girl, Makeela, with a neck injury. I introduced myself to her mother. She spoke in a rich African accent. She said, "Makeela fell and hurt her neck."

Her accent reminded me of Nigeria, "Where are you from, originally?"

She smiled warmly, her teeth brilliant against her dark skin, "We're from Ghana. We've been in the U.S. about three years."

"I worked at a hospital in Nigeria in medical school for a few months. I'd like to go back someday; I learned a lot there."

She asked, "What did you learn?"

I said, "I learned tropical medicine and African culture. I also learned about contentment."

One of the benefits of travel is being able to connect. When I meet an Arab patient, I often say, "I've been to the Middle East. The people are so friendly." Tensions seem to melt.

In Nigeria, the moment that impacted me most was visiting a leper village. The people had been kicked out of their villages for being lepers and lived in abject poverty. Most were horribly disfigured, missing digits and parts of their faces. They would burn grass and club mice and rats that ran out. We saw them roasting rats on an open fire—rat on a stick.

They invited us to a worship service at the lone church. One of the members led singing. Since they were from different tribes, English was the common language. They sang as if the louder and more pure their voices, the better God would hear.

The leader asked, "Who has God blessed the most?" The entire congregation erupted with cheering and laughing, "Me! God has blessed me the most!" They smiled and clapped.

I looked at Missy and she smiled through tears. We have talked about that moment over and over. Their contentment and thankfulness were humbling. I can get annoyed when the grocery line is too long.

Makeela's mother said wistfully, "You should go to Ghana, it's very beautiful. I miss it."

I examined Makeela's neck and saw a harsh purple abrasion that wrapped from the front of her throat to the back of her neck, almost a perfect circle, except a few inches on the right side where there was no abrasion. I was baffled and concerned.

"How did this happen?"

"She told me that she fell off an exercise bike in our family room. I think she may have hit the bike when she fell."

"I see. We'll take an X-ray of her neck and make sure she hasn't injured the bones."

I walked out of the room with a pit in my insides. I could not imagine how the injury could have been caused by anything except an attempted strangulation. It looked like a cord or wire had been wrapped around the child's neck and squeezed with murderous intent, enough to break the skin and bruise the underlying tissue.

Whoever did this was not a nice person.

I called one of my partners for a second opinion. "Mike, could you come to the pediatric area? I'm seeing a little girl who has an injury suspicious for child abuse."

We examined her together, and then walked out of the room. I asked, "Can you think of anything besides child abuse that could cause that injury?"

"No. I guess you'll have to call Child Protective Services. Her mom seems really nice."

"Yeah, it's hard to believe she'd be involved in abuse."

I looked at the X-ray. I knew what I had to do, but I didn't want to. I dreaded returning to the room. Child abuse would be an incredibly sad situation. If it weren't abuse, she might feel falsely accused. The situation was more complex since they were immigrants. I stared blankly at the normal X-ray and mustered the will to talk with her mother.

I walked in and said, "Her X-ray looks fine. Who was with your daughter when this happened?"

"No one. My husband was in the next room, in his office. He heard her fall. She ran toward the kitchen where I was. There was no one else in the house."

I said, "I don't understand how this happened by falling off a stationary bicycle. It looks like something was wrapped around her neck."

"I know. I don't know how that happened."

"Do you think your husband might have disciplined her by wrapping something around her neck?"

"No. He's a gentle father and loves his little girl."

I swallowed, "I have to report this. Someone will come tonight to investigate. We need to get to the bottom of this."

Her face was peaceful, "That's all right. I want what's best for her and I understand your concern. My husband wouldn't do this. He's been a patient father with our two older children."

"Where were the other children?"

"At a neighbor's house."

"I want to make this as easy as possible for your family. Can you call your husband and ask him to come? It'll be helpful to talk with him."

About an hour later, I saw Makeela's father—wearing a colorful African robe—arrive with both sons. Makeela beamed and shouted "Daddy!" and hugged his leg. He put his big hand on her back and hugged her.

It did not add up. All types of people abuse children, and appearances can be deceptive, but she seemed happy with both parents. Maybe they were protecting someone else?

The investigator from Child Protective Services and a police officer arrived. She asked about the case.

I said, "The injuries don't fit with falling off an exercise bike. It looks like someone tried to strangle her.

"Her parents seem mild-mannered and sweet. Her father arrived a few minutes ago; she ran over and gave him a big hug. She's too young to fake it."

The CPS officer interviewed the family. Thirty minutes later she came out. "We're going with the family now to investigate the scene. The police officer will go with me. I'll call you after the investigation."

I went back to work feeling uneasy.

⊞ ⊞ ⊞

The next patient, Sunshine, was a 6-year-old with a fever. Her mother had braided long hair, no makeup, and wore a hemp cloth dress. She was polite, but I thought she had a glint of distrust in her eyes. She introduced her five other children: Echo, Promise, Jasmine, Tree, and Luna. They were all under ten years old and had bright blonde hair.

In taking the history, I asked, "Are Sunshine's vaccinations up to date?"

She said, "No, we love our kids too much to subject them to that."

"What do you mean?"

"My husband and I believe in doing everything naturally and living our lives in harmony with the earth. We don't believe in putting unnecessary chemicals in our children's bodies."

"Are you worried about autism? I know there has been concern that vaccinations could cause autism. A huge study recently showed—without a doubt—autism is not caused by vaccinations."

"Who did the study? Western doctors?"

"I suppose there were doctors involved. The study showed there were no differences between autism rates in vaccinated versus unvaccinated children. The main difference with unvaccinated children is they're much more likely to die from preventable causes." I hated to be so blunt.

Her eyes flashed, "My natural healer said that this would happen if I brought Sunshine to the ER. You should read the book, 'What Your Doctor Failed to Mention.'"

Time to change the subject.

"How long has Sunshine been sick?"

"Her fever began last week. My holistic practitioner prescribed herbal remedies and advised aromatherapy and energy work. She was getting better but now she's vomiting the elixir."

"Has she had abdominal pain?"

"She said her belly hurt, but we did a few cleansing enemas to rid the body of unnatural toxins. That helped."

"O.K., I will look her over." I examined Sunshine; she wore a clean simple dress and looked at me nervously. I tried to reassure her by smiling and asking about school.

Her eyes settled too deep and her lips were parched—she was dehydrated. When I palpated her abdomen, she grimaced.

"I'm worried about her abdomen. She could have appendicitis."

"I want to be informed of the risks before Sunny is exposed to any radiation or toxic medicines. But do what you think is right; that's why we are here."

"We should do a CAT scan, it's the best test for appendicitis. There is radiation that could theoretically have negative heath effects, but in her case, the risk of not doing surgery could be fatal."

"I need to call my husband and my healing practitioner."

"I'd be glad to talk with either."

    ⊡ ⊡ ⊡

Caleb was a cherub with a mop of blonde hair. The 3-year-old had fallen and bitten through his tongue.

Sewing a tongue is tricky business, like holding a slippery eel. The tongue has to be anchored. I took a suturing needle and pierced the tongue, about a half-inch from the tip. I ran nylon thread through and secured it in a clamp that an assistant held. The traction of the stitch held the tongue outside of the mouth. The boy looked like a dead deer on the roadside, his tongue completely out of his mouth and pulled to one side.

I could feel the horrified mother's eyes boring a hole into the side of my head as I sutured the tongue.

Caleb didn't seem to mind much. I gave him a sucker and a Spiderman sticker afterward, and we were friends for life.

⬛ ⬛ ⬛

I went back to talk with Sunshine's mother. She agreed to the CAT scan.

A few minutes later the Child Protective Services worker called, "We went to the room where the injury happened. Makeela ran to the stationary bike and said, 'I was climbing up here and this was around my neck. I fell off.' Beside the bike, there was a closed loop string that adjusts a window blind. Does this fit with the nature of her injuries?"

I felt the weight lift. I replied, "That makes sense. I wondered why she would have a harsh abrasion around three fourths of her neck and the rest appear untouched."

She said, "They seem like nice people. We consider this case closed."

I was relieved. I hoped Makeela's family would not have negative feelings.

We see children with injuries almost every shift. We are required by law to report any suspicion of child abuse. I hate to call CPS on an innocent family whose child has an accident. Even worse is not reporting a family where serious abuse is occurring. We often see obvious cases; the tricky ones are vague and unclear.

We see psychiatric patients who were horribly sexually and physically abused as children. The scary converse is that we unknowingly see many children who are being abused, and they leave the ER with a sucker and a Spiderman sticker—back to the hell of abuse.

◨　◨　◨

I went to look up something in a textbook in our office. One of my older partners was dictating. I told him about Sunshine. He pulled off his reading glasses and rubbed his gray beard. He said, "They want to do everything naturally? Natural is what life was like two hundred years ago, or in places where there's no access to modern medical care. Natural is dying at forty years of age, which is what life expectancy used to be, and still is in parts of the world. Natural is dying during childbirth. Natural is dying from appendicitis. Of course, it's fine if that is how they want to live, but why pretend natural is always more healthy."

I said, "Yeah, Sunshine is not looking very healthy now. Maybe natural by the definition you just gave, but she is not the picture of health. I feel sorry for her mother, as I'm sure she's trying to do what's best, but I'm worried that she may've waited too long. I think her appendix may've burst."

He said, "I'm a product of the sixties, sort of a leftist hippy, and this bothers me for the same reason my mother would get irked at sham preachers—she thought they were giving true faith a bad name. I heard about Jimmy Swaggart for years after that debacle. Non-medical healing reminds me of faith healers. Sort of like right-wing nut jobs and left-wing nut jobs: two sides of the same coin. Both sides appeal to people who are antiestablishment and distrustful of society."

I said, "I had a patient in residency who refused blood and died."

"Jehovah's Witness?"

"Yeah."

He said, "That's living your faith. Or I guess, dying for your faith. Don't get me wrong; I'm not harshing on spirituality. I respect prayer, yoga, meditation, whatever. But there's a difference between providing spiritual support and deceiving your followers. Most of these practitioners probably believe it, but that doesn't make it work. That family might not call their beliefs a religion, but that's pretty much what it is.

"Some people don't like change or progress. They pine for the good old days: both religious fundamentalists and Earth worshipers. Busybodies at my mother's church told her using pain meds during childbirth was a sin because the Bible says childbirth should be painful. She told them, 'If you'd mind your own business, you wouldn't have time to mind mine.'" He laughed and said, "She was a tough old gal."

He continued, "If you want to be healthy: eat natural whole foods, exercise, get enough sleep, spend time outdoors, drink in moderation, avoid fast food, don't smoke, don't shoot heroin."

I said, "But don't you think people have a right to do what they want with their health or bodies?"

He said, "Of course. But there's scientific truth that's beyond the realm of the mystical. If you don't have surgery on your appendix, it is not good, no matter what you believe about it."

I went back to work. An hour later I got a call from the radiologist, "Your patient, Sunshine Jones, has a ruptured appendix. There are multiple abscesses throughout her abdomen. The largest one is four centimeters in diameter."

I dreaded telling her mother the news because I hate giving bad news to patients, especially about children, and I felt like it would be a slap in the face to her beliefs—a double whammy. Sort of like saying: you have cancer AND God doesn't hear your prayers.

I told her mother the news, "The CAT scan shows that she has appendicitis; unfortunately her appendix has burst."

She asked, "What does that mean?"

"She needs surgery. After the appendix bursts, it spills bacteria into the abdomen. The bacteria causes infections that will not heal on their own, they have to be surgically drained. One abscess is larger than a golf ball. She'll be in the hospital for several days on IV antibiotics. Her abdominal wound has to be left open to heal from the bottom. If they close after surgery, the abscess will form again. She'll have to be out of school for a few weeks."

She said, "I want to talk with my practitioner. I'm not sure I agree with your plan. Isn't there a non-surgical, more natural approach?"

I thought, if she were in rural Africa, natural would be the only option.

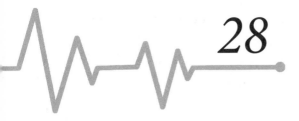

28

Ten days later, I looked up Sunshine. Her parents eventually agreed to surgery. Sunny was still in the hospital with an open abdominal wound. She had gotten very sick after surgery with high fevers and vomiting. She had to have a repeat CAT scan to see if the abscess had returned. She was still unable to eat and was on IV fluids.

I wondered what her mother thought, as she seemed to consider modern, Western medicine the enemy. She had spent the last week and a half living behind enemy lines. I wondered if her views had changed, or if she considered the ordeal a necessary evil. Surgery, antibiotics, IV fluids: none of it is natural, but neither are clothes or running water.

Her mother wanted what was best for Sunny, and tried to do the right thing. We are all products of our upbringing, personalities, and experiences; judging her would be shallow.

▣ ▣ ▣

Noah met multiple times with his lawyer to prepare for the lawsuit. The lead lawyer was a surgeon's son and passionate about defending doctors.

Noah spent most of his days preparing for the case. I had not seen him much. He was trying not to be consumed by the trial, but seemed to be losing the battle.

They were suing for six million dollars. The malpractice

insurance only covered up to three million. If the jury awarded their request, Noah would start out his career three million dollars in the hole. That would be on top of the one hundred and fifty thousand he owed for med school: three million, one hundred and fifty thousand dollars.

After meeting with his lawyer, he stopped by my house. We sat on the front porch.

He said, "My lawyer, Reggie, is cool, but I hate sitting around in his stuffy leather and mahogany office. This is sucking all my free time. I haven't been outside much in weeks.

"Reggie said the plaintiff's lawyer wouldn't have taken the case if they didn't think they could win. He thinks it'll be hard to defend.

"There's some controversy in the cardiology literature about whether delayed cath or a clot-busting drug is more beneficial. It's clear that heart cath is better than CB normally, but it's not clear in delayed cases.

"You aren't going to believe this—they have a local ER doctor who's never testified in a case before. He's going to take the stand and say I committed malpractice."

I said, "You're kidding me! Someone from Portland?"

He grimaced, "Yep. They also have a second physician witness: a hired gun from out of town, but he'll have limited credibility since he's testified multiple times against doctors. Reggie's dealt with him before and said he's fairly easy to discredit.

"The first doctor sounds like an ace in the hole for them. Reggie's guess is that he's the backbone of their entire case; without him, this would be a weak case and the med mal firm would judge it too weak to pursue. Having this doctor is a rainmaker for them and a doom-bringer for us. They're spending mucho pesos to litigate this.

"The best thing for us is that Hans Maier's going to testify on my behalf. Reggie said that he commands respect due to his stature and the fact that he's such a distinguished, handsome speaker. Juries love him."

I said, "I bet they do; that guy oozes charisma. I always felt fortunate to have him as our residency director. That's huge!"

"Yeah, I was stoked. Reggie said Dr. Maier will decline to witness if it's obvious malpractice, but in most of the cases he's the star witness. Did you hear his talk on lawsuits during residency?"

"Yeah. He saw me commit malpractice during residency when I over-sedated that guy with a shoulder dislocation. Did Reggie have any idea who their witness is? I can't believe someone from Portland would testify."

"No, we don't know yet. I have a feeling it may be someone who recently moved here and isn't well connected. There are three older guys in Gresham who recently came from California. Reggie thinks it's one of them. They'll have to identify their witnesses before the trial so we'll know. Reggie said he's worried about this person. A credible emergency doctor from our community will be very influential to a jury—likely enough to sink us."

He tried to put on a brave face, but I knew him too well. He was scared.

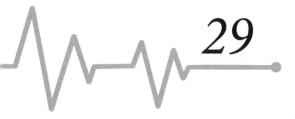

29

A few weeks later, Noah pulled up to my house. I loaded my mountain bike. We picked up coffee and headed out of town to meet a buddy at the Lewis River trail, near Mount St Helens.

I asked, "What's up with the trial?"

He said, "Nothing new. This is my first day in a month to do something fun."

"How're you feeling about it?"

"My lawyer said we probably have a forty percent chance of winning. He thinks that if we lose, the full six million was a likely verdict. Mr. Bristol's lost wages for the rest of his career are calculated to be over five million. He's a big-time banker. Toss in pain and suffering and six million seems reasonable."

"How're you doing?"

"Some days I'm fine. Some days I'm far, far from fine."

He was driving and I looked at him. His jaw was tight and his eyes narrowed. I was sad to see such a happy guy brought low.

I said, "I'm sure it will be O.K."

"If you call a sixty percent chance and three million dollars debt O.K."

We drove on in silence for a few minutes. He said, "Let's don't talk about this with Eric. I need a break from the drama."

We pulled in to the trailhead and Eric was waiting for us. He was one of my partners at Brookwood. He was a little older; a cool, sporty guy. He bore a remarkable likeness to Mark Green from the television show ER. Once, a camera crew from a Portland television station followed him around and made a big deal about how much he looked like Mark Green.

Eric said, "Check out this, I saw a patient who'd been eating bento chicken on a wooden skewer while driving. He'd rear-ended another car and his airbag deployed. The airbag drove the skewer through his hand, tongue, and both cheeks. He arrived in the ER with his hand stapled to his face—palm outward—by the skewer; his mouth forced in an O. Chicken was on the skewer sticking out of his palm.

"He couldn't talk; he looked like he had been attacked by an elf with a bow and arrow. We gave him morphine and I jerked the skewer out with pliers. Even after the skewer was removed, he held his mouth in an O."

Noah said, "Dude. That is freaked out."

I asked, "How did it get his hand also?"

Eric said, "He probably dropped it during the crash and all of it was crunched together when the airbag exploded. He had surgery on his hand."

I said, "I was about to do a pelvic exam on a patient. Her feet were up in the stirrups and a sheet was draped over her legs.

"I went to sit on the wheeled stool and missed the center. I had the speculum in my hands. The stool rolled backward; I was in a squatting position about to sit. I started stumbling backward in a squatting position and the stool rolled away from me. The stool crashed into the wall and I sat on it abruptly.

"The nurse was at the head of the bed. The patient couldn't see what happened, but I'm sure she wondered what the clatter was about. I raised my eyebrows in a 'Wow. That was a close one' expression. The nurse started shaking, trying not to laugh. You know how it's much funnier when you aren't supposed to laugh?

I quit looking at the nurse in order to regain my composure, but I almost burst out laughing. I don't think the patient ever knew what happened."

We rode a little farther and then stopped at an overlook. The bright teal water flowed below, weaving among massive old growth firs. We sat on moss-covered rocks.

Not to be outdone, Noah said, "Here's a tale you haven't heard before. When I was in high school, I was driving home after missing my curfew. I was going to be grounded and I was angry. I opened the moon roof in my car. I put the car on cruise control at about seventy miles an hour and then stood up in the seat. I sat on the roof of the car and steered with my feet."

I said, "You're lying! You didn't do that! You could've been killed so easily."

He laughed, "I ain't lying and I didn't die."

Eric said, "Here's my weirdest ER story. This happened at Brookwood." He told us this story.

◨　◧　◨

Eric was sewing up a lac on an elderly woman's head when he saw a commotion. The nurses wheeled back a bloody young man on a stretcher. Eric saw a small squirt of blood shoot from his chest with each heartbeat. He quickly excused himself and ran out of the patient's room.

Eric asked, "What happened?"

A nurse said, "He was stabbed and his friends drove him here. His name is Blake; he's sixteen."

"Where are his friends?"

"In the waiting room."

At Brookwood, we hardly ever see stab wounds. The only stabbings we see are patients brought by private vehicles; ambulances take them to the trauma center.

Eric said, "Bring his friends back. Blake, what happened?"

"Some guy downtown stabbed me. We weren't doing anything wrong; some random guy just stuck me with a knife."

"Were you stabbed more than once? Were you hurt in any other way?"

"No, he just stabbed me in the chest and ran off."

"Any shortness of breath?"

"No, but it hurts to take a deep breath."

Eric said to the nurses, "Set up for a chest tube. Order a stat portable chest X-ray. I need the ultrasound machine."

Eric quickly examined Blake. He had a single stab wound to the left lower part of his chest, near his sternum. A small spray of blood squirted with each heartbeat, like an automatic lawn sprinkler.

The nurse shouted, "Blood pressure normal, 130 systolic. Heart rate is 110." The nurses started an IV on each arm.

Anticipating that this could go south quickly, Eric said, "Please get a respiratory therapist and bring intubation equipment."

The two friends were brought back. They were normal appearing high school students; they looked frightened.

Eric asked, "What happened?"

One of them said, "Some dude just ran up to Blake and stabbed him and ran off."

The other said, "Tell the truth! It's not the time to lie!"

The first one glanced around anxiously as if the police were watching, "You won't tell our parents, or the cops?"

Eric replied, "Tell me what happened. We need the whole story."

"We wanted to try snorting coke. We'd never done that before. Blake heard that if you ask around on Burnside, it's pretty easy to score. A creepy looking dude said that he'd sell us some, and led us into a dark alley. When Blake handed him the two hundred dollars, the guy counted it, then he reached into his coat, and in one motion pulled out a knife and stabbed Blake. Just like, 'Pow!" Blake dropped to the ground and the guy ran off. We grabbed Blake, ran for the car, and drove here."

Eric said, "Get cardiothoracic surgery on the phone, stat. This may involve his heart. Bring in a central line kit. Run two liters of normal saline wide open. Send off routine blood work, a blood count, electrolytes, and a cross match for his blood type."

"Am I going to die? That guy tried to kill me! He must have missed my heart? Right?"

"We will see. The fact that your vital signs are almost normal is a good sign."

"I can't believe this happened to me. I mean I was like…" His words trailed off into a slur and he passed out.

Eric yelled, "Blake!"

No reply. "Bring the ultrasound! Set up for a thoracotomy! We need to crack his chest!"

The nurse yelled, "I can't feel a pulse! I don't think he has a blood pressure!"

Eric squirted ultrasound gel and slapped the probe on his chest. He could see that the sack around his heart, the pericardium, was full of blood. The heart was not beating well. Normally the stiff fibrous sack is lubricated with a trace of fluid and the heart beats inside the sack. The pericardial sack protects the heart from rubbing directly on the lungs and sternum. When it is full of blood, the stiff sack can't expand and puts pressure on the heart. The heart will be squeezed to the point of being unable to expand. This is known as pericardial tamponade.

Blake's heart was like a man in quicksand. The heart struggled against the liquid straightjacket that held it, but the harder the heart fought, the tighter the trap grew.

With tamponade, the blood pressure will suddenly drop, blood ceases to flow to the rest of the body, and the patient will die—unless something is done quickly.

The blood had stopped flowing from Blake's heart into his body; his body and brain were dying.

Often pericardial tamponade can be drained with a needle under the sternum. In Blake's case, his chest needed to be opened because the blood would refill the pericardium immediately due to the hole in his heart. The hole needed to be repaired to stop the flow of blood into the pericardial sack. Quickly.

Eric intubated Blake and moved to the chest. He put on a gown and mask.

One of his friends—his face like skim milk—mumbled in shock, "Oh, no. No. Please. No."

The other was crying, tears rolling down his teenaged cheeks. "He's dead! My best friend is dead! We were going to be college roommates and now he's dead!" He let out a sob.

Eric muttered, "Not yet he isn't. Not just yet."

He poured cleaning solution on Blake's chest and yanked a scalpel off the tray. He placed the scalpel on his chest and cut between two ribs over his entombed heart. He cut through skin and muscle and could see a sliver of the heart between the ribs. He placed rib spreaders between the ribs and cranked them open. He saw the heart—a violet quivering ball. Blake's youthful heart struggled against the incarceration.

He cut into the pericardium with scissors. When he nicked the pericardium, clotted blood punched out like a purple arm. He lengthened the incision, a gelatinous blob fell out, and he scooped the blood with his hand. The heart—freed from the liquid tomb—beat vigorously and triumphantly.

Blake moved. They had not paralyzed and sedated him because he was dead when they started.

He was no longer dead. Blood was arriving fast and furious to his body and brain.

"Give him one hundred milligrams of succ and twenty of etomidate. I don't want him to move." We paralyzed him

He searched the heart for the site of the bleeding. He saw blood flowing out, but was unable to see the source.

"Suction please."

The nurse placed a suction catheter into his gloved hand. He suctioned the blood.

He could see blood leaking from the muscle of the heart.

"Nylon stitch on a needle driver." The nurse slapped his palm with the needle driver. He held the curved needle above the muscle of the heart where blood was flowing. The heart was beating: thump-thump, thump-thump. He hesitated for the pause between beats and nailed it on the first attempt. He tied the stitch off; no blood escaped. Blake's—and Eric's—heart beat vigorously.

"Call the University. We have a trauma transfer." He placed a drain into the area around his heart and removed the rib spreaders. He loosely stitched the chest shut. Eric took the call and talked with the trauma surgeon at the University.

He hung up and told the nurses, "They are sending the helicopter so they don't have to worry about traffic. They will be here in fifteen minutes."

Eric looked at Blake's friends. They were gray, but the relief shone from their faces.

"Is he going to be all right?"

"I think so. He'll have the final repair in the operating room at the University."

The helicopter arrived and whisked him away.

⊡ ⊡ ⊡

Noah was throwing rocks into the river below. He said, "What happened to him?"

"He was fine. In fact, he came to the ER a few months later to thank us. He was running track and talking about college."

I said, "That was a save. You jumped in the deep water and pulled out a drowning man."

"Yeah, I was pretty stoked. Times like that make this job worth it."

Noah and I made eye contact. He shrugged his shoulders as if he were not sure. I smiled sadly.

The next time I saw Eric, I received a wrenching shock.

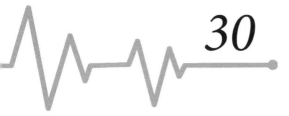

30

A few weeks later, we were having a routine evening in the ER. I was enjoying myself, working with some of my favorite staff.

A tech greeted me, "It's the sexy man boy! What's up SMB?" I smiled. I have been called SMB ever since I met Tuan.

Thanks, Tuan.

I interviewed a mentally ill patient. He had spent time in prison for sexual assault. His teeth looked burnt and there was food in his beard. He oozed the foul scent of stale cigarettes, dirty underclothes, and yuck mouth. I asked, "Why are you here today, sir?"

He said, "I can't deny myself any longer. I want to rape as many people as possible."

I repressed a shudder. I couldn't think of a proper question. I asked, "Who do you want to rape?"

"I mostly like to rape children." He smiled, his dark teeth cemented with yellowish ick.

Something inside me turned. Twisted. Sprang to life. I felt my eyes widen, letting in more darkness. I wanted to charge him, clutch his throat in my needy hands, and squeeze. I wanted, needed, to throttle the obscene smile off his face.

I twitched, "Why did you come to the ER?"

"Because I don't want to keep raping. I like it, but I don't want to go to hell." His tongue ran across his chapped lips.

My heart slammed against my ribs like a prisoner banging on jail bars. The thing inside of me wanted to get out, to kill the thing inside him. It pounded. Banged.

I could not wait to escape his presence. I rushed out before the insanity flowed between us.

I told security, "Kill him if he tries to leave."

They laughed. I did not.

I spoke with a social worker about the patient, and we put him on a hold, taking away his ability to leave voluntarily. The social worker hoped we could get him involuntarily committed to the state hospital.

I hoped also. I really hoped. That man should not be allowed in public ever, ever again.

I saw a few more patients. I saw an elderly man who was more confused than usual, a young woman with a migraine, a middle aged man with a nosebleed who was on blood thinners, and an infant with a fever.

Beth was the next patient, a 25-year-old who probably weighed four hundred pounds.

Beth had abdominal pain. I was concerned; massively overweight people are hard to diagnose. A physical exam is difficult. She would not fit in a CAT scanner. Drawing blood might not be possible.

The average lifespan of someone her size is around forty years of age. Their problems are notoriously hard to diagnose and treat.

I shook hands with Beth and her mother; they were both polite. Her mother was thin.

Beth was so mammoth that she crossed her arms across her chest to keep her arms from hanging off the bed. She had a shy smile, like a child. She didn't appear to be in discomfort. I asked, "What is your problem today?"

Her mother replied, "Her stomach hurts."

I asked Beth, "Where does your abdomen hurt?"

Her mother replied, "In the lower part."

I asked Beth, "When did this start?"

She looked at her mom, who replied, "She started feeling it about two days ago, but it's worse today."

I saw that I was dealing with an overprotective parent who acted as if her adult child was a helpless toddler. When I took psychiatry in med school they explained a dynamic I've seen play out multiple times. Overbearing parents become deeply involved in their child's life. They treat the child as helpless. They spoon-feed the child who is much too old.

As the child gets older, an unconscious dilemma is faced: "What will happen when I become an adult and leave the house?" This thought is deeply disturbing. The subconscious solution is to become obese, therefore never separating from the parents. It also works for the parents; they keep their baby at home and worry over them.

"Have you had any vomiting or fever?"

Her mom said, "No, she hasn't."

I heard yelling. I looked out—Mr. Freak Nasty Rape was making his break. He was running full speed down the hallway toward me with a security guard in pursuit. The security guard had been escorting him to the restroom when he bolted.

I was in a side room that entered into the hall. He was running down the hall and would run past in a moment. His face had a look of blissful anticipation—a hungry creature eager to feed.

I eased from my seat and paused. He was close. I waited.

Game on.

I dropped my hips and shoulders, rushed three steps, and exploded into him with every bit of high school enthusiasm I had in my non-high school body. I came from the side and he didn't see me until the last moment. He did not have time to react. I struck him from the side like a linebacker hitting a surprised, outstretched receiver. I straightened my hips and knees, and threw my weight.

He spun sideways and horizontally—I think his shoulder and head struck the ground before the rest of him. His head sounded like a bowling ball clunking the floor. His breath hissed explosively through charred teeth, spraying foul spittle.

I crouched over him, wanting to touch His Nastiness as little as possible. The security guards piled on. He groaned and moaned, and groaned some more.

I picked up my stethoscope, chart, and papers, but what I really wanted to do was stand with fists raised above my head like I had sacked the quarterback. I longed to lean down and poke my finger in his face with a taunting grin. "Don't think you can run the ball up in here. Not against this defense. No sir! Bad for your health!" I could have spiked my prescription pad, twirled my stethoscope above my head, and high stepped down the hall in a victory dance.

I restrained myself.

Mr. Malodorous Sicko Perv was returned to his room and the door was locked. Fortunately—I guess—he was unhurt by our little embrace.

Later one of my partners, Dave, said, "Nice job on the gentle patient restraint. I'm glad to hear you treat all your patients with loving kindness."

I laughed, "If I was in better shape, I would've picked him up and dropped him on his head. Did you hear why he was here?"

"Yes. The nurses were talking about him. Sounds like a real piece of work. Have you heard the story about my patient restraint?"

"No. Tell me."

❏   ❏   ❏

Dave and Pablo, a nurse, were in the break room, drinking coffee and chatting. They heard yelling coming from the ER and ran into the hall. A disheveled man in his mid-thirties was walking rapidly toward them. He wore a dirty trench coat and dark boots. He had a greenish tattoo on his cheek, bald on his skullcap, and his hair hung in unhealthy strands down his long neck. He held a large butcher knife in his hand.

Sue, a nurse, was following him. Sue shouted, "He says he's going to slaughter the nurses on the psychiatric ward! He walked so fast through the ER that no one noticed him! I don't think security knows! That's Carl Tate! He said he's going to gouge their eyes out!"

Carl walked briskly toward Dave, ignoring Sue. He was holding the knife next to his waist, pointed down and slightly outward. The blade edge was forward.

Dave said, "Get security! Call the police! Call the psych ward!" Sue turned and ran back toward the ER.

Pablo and Dave stepped into the break room, out of his way. Carl moved past and did not look in.

Carl Tate was well known to the ER at Brookwood. He was one of the worst players that visited regularly. He had a rage syndrome and a personality disorder. He didn't have schizophrenia, just seething fury. He was seen in the ER the previous year after he had ruined a poor child's day.

The 7-year-old was playing with her pet bunny rabbit in a leafy neighborhood park. Her mother was reading a book on a park bench. Carl grabbed the bunny by the nape, and sunk his teeth into the rabbit's neck. The mother scooped up her child and ran away. He followed behind, sucking and chewing on the rabbit with blood dripping from his chin, while the child watched in horror over her mother's shoulder.

He spent time on the psychiatric ward after that and may have gone to jail.

He was back.

After he walked by, Pablo stepped out to follow. Carl was thirty feet in front, rapidly walking down a long back hallway.

Dave ran back to the ER to see where the security personnel were; he saw none. He yelled to a nurse, "Get security to the back hallway! Now!"

He turned around and ran toward the hallway. He saw Pablo and Carl ahead. He was about one hundred feet behind, thinking about the best course of action. They had to stop him before he made it to the stairs or met someone else coming toward him; he might slash anyone.

Pablo is small, but gritty, and Dave is big: they could probably overpower Carl, but it would be dangerous. They had no weapons; there was nothing in the barren hallway they could use.

Pablo said, "Carl, where are you going?" His voice echoed down the long, wide hallway. Carl ignored Pablo and kept walking.

Dave tried to think of a way to cut him off, or to thwart his forward motion.

Pablo yelled, "Carl, stop!"

Carl peered over his shoulder; then he turned his gaze forward and walked at a brisk clip.

He suddenly spun and ran toward Pablo. He held the knife out to the side. He made a feral moan.

Pablo turned and ran away. Pablo could outrun him, but he maintained the thirty feet distance. He was courageously keeping him close.

Dave stepped into a side hallway. He flattened his back to the edge of the corner, with his head turned toward the larger, main hallway.

Pablo rushed by, looking over his shoulder. He saw Dave, but didn't acknowledge.

Carl came into view, his yellow teeth bared, his marble eyes narrowed.

212

Dave pivoted and threw his weight into his forearm.

Clothesline.

His forearm struck Carl in his nose. Carl's knees buckled, and he toppled backward.

Dave put both hands on the arm with the knife, then pinned Carl's hand with his knee.

Pablo rushed up, grabbed Carl's legs, and lay across his lower body.

Dave rocked forward, putting most of his weight on his knee. Carl released the knife. Dave tossed it down the hallway with a clatter. Carl didn't try to fight. He just lay looking stunned. He let out a long involuntary groan; his breath had been knocked out. His eyes glazed.

Less than one minute later, a crew of security guards clamored down the hallway. They heaped on and held him down.

A few nurses rushed down with a stretcher. They lifted him and tied him down with restraints.

◨   ◨   ◨

I said, "Wow. That was a close one. What were you thinking when you were about to hit him?"

"I don't remember. It was all pretty instinctual."

"Yeah, that's how I felt with the Grim Raper. That was pretty brave of Pablo."

"I was impressed by how he played cat-and-mouse perfectly."

"What happened to Carl?"

"He went to jail. He was ordered by the judge to never return to Brookwood, so I'm not sure where he is now. He used to come here often, but that was the last time."

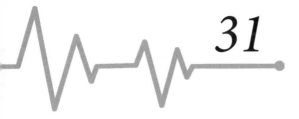

31

We stopped skiing. We sat on a slope to take a break and admire the view. It was Tuesday and we had the place to ourselves. Snow loaded the branches of the high alpine fir trees. The clouds boiled in the valley below, pouring chowder over Portland. We rose above and enjoyed the sun.

Noah said, "Now this is the way to escape the Portland rain."

I said, "I love coming up here. Listen to this, I waylaid a pervert trying to bolt from the ER." I told him the story.

He said, "Did you tackle him harder than you would have a regular psych patient who was trying to escape?"

"For sure. I would have just arm tackled or grabbed a regular patient. In my defense, that guy has a violent past. He needed to be taken out of commission. He might have bitten someone during the takedown or something. His teeth carried the rot of ages."

"Sounds like a good justification, tough guy. Were you proud of yourself?"

I smiled, "Maybe."

"Watch out Cranky the Clown, here comes Dr. Tough Guy Russell off the top rope!"

I stared at Mount Jefferson in the distance, a twin of Mount Hood. I hated to ask, but hated not to, "What's the latest with the lawsuit?"

Noah said, "We talk about every angle and every possible question. Even when we're not meeting, I think about it. It's always with me, like a cancer. Today, I'm even thinking about it when I'm snowboarding."

"This, too, shall pass."

"True, but millions of dollars of debt will be with me for a mighty long time: the gift that keeps giving, like an STD." He pulled his water bottle out of his backpack. "What's the difference between true love and herpes?"

"What?"

"Love is temporary, herpes is forever."

I winced, "I diagnosed a woman with her first outbreak of herpes on her fortieth wedding anniversary. The exact day! Her husband looked so guilty. He got caught with his hand in the nookie jar."

"That's horrible. That guy is The Scarlet Letterman. He should be castrated."

He took a swig from his water bottle and said, "I wish I were able to deal with the stress more positively. It's consuming me. I lie awake thinking about it. I wake up thinking about it. I'm getting less sleep. I think I'm depressed. I can't believe I'm being sued for trying my hardest. I can't believe I'm being sued without making a mistake. Mostly, I can't believe a local doctor is testifying against me."

"That's unbelievable: Dr. Judas Iscariot."

"I'm sure whomever it is will be paid more than thirty pieces of silver."

"How are things at home?"

"Suzie and I are arguing more. I want to be left alone, but when I'm alone the dread overwhelms me. It drives me mad that I'm letting the stress affect my personal life. She wants everything to be hunky dory. I know I bring stress home more than I used to, but I wish she'd get off my back."

"I thought you guys were bulletproof. I can't imagine you arguing much."

"I thought so, too. She seems to think I can have massive stress at work and this trial hanging over my head and come home all smiles and roses. I wish that were the case, but it's not realistic."

I said, "I know most ER doctors get sued, but for you to get sued so soon after residency, for such a weak reason, is brutal. It's bringing me down, but I'm sure it's much worse for you. I'm so sorry you are going through this."

He clamored to his feet. "Whatever. I'll survive. That which doesn't kill me, almost does. I bet I can beat you to the bottom."

He pointed his snowboard downhill, but I was ready. I pushed off with my poles and got the jump on him.

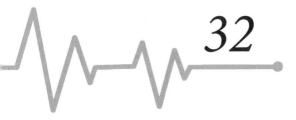

32

A few days later, I was reading a novel at home. A minute later, I heard Missy's cell phone ring; she talked frantically. She ran down the stairs, and burst into the room.

"Here's Brent. I'll give the phone to him." She thrust the phone toward me, "It's Marge! She says Eric's had a stroke!" I took the phone.

Marge said, "Brent, I think Eric had a stroke. He's totally unresponsive."

I said, "Call 911. I'll be there in two minutes."

I ran out of the house and jumped into my car; I broke every traffic law as I sped the half-mile to Eric's house. He had a stroke? That did not make sense. Forty-three-year-old athletes with no medical problems do not have strokes. I had ridden mountain bikes with Noah and him a few weeks earlier. He ran marathons. We had recently traveled together to Baja, Mexico on a windsurfing trip. Eric and Noah were the star windsurfers. Maybe he blew a brain aneurysm. I shuddered at the thought.

I slammed the car into park and bolted into the house. Their two girls, seven and ten, were huddled together looking as if they'd seen a ghost. Eric was on the floor, unresponsive, his gaze horribly blank. Marge was tearful, but controlled, "He was fine. We were having dinner and he became unresponsive. He was talking to me, then he slurred his words, and then went silent." She held her hand over her mouth, her eyes brimming.

Eric stared at the ceiling. I felt his neck for a pulse; it felt strong. I shook his shoulders, "Eric! Eric!" He seemed to see me for a moment and then faded. He had a drugged, stuporous look. Maybe he had a seizure?

I noticed margarita glasses on the table. "How much did he drink tonight?"

"I think he had two margaritas. We were in the middle of dinner and were having a coherent conversation. He was talking, his words slurred suddenly, and then he blanked. He was far from drunk."

I asked "Did he take any medicine?"

At my medical school, an anesthesiology resident came in the ER after being seriously injured in a car accident. When his clothes were cut off, a central line was discovered, sewed into his groin. He was abusing IV narcotics that he was stealing from the OR.

Marge replied, "No. I'm positive."

Marge huddled with a daughter under each arm. All three were crying. My pulse thundered.

I grabbed his shoulders and squeezed. He looked into my eyes and slowly blinked. I said, "Eric! Can you hear me?" His head rolled and he breathed heavily, a trickle of drool escaped his lips. His eyes closed.

I did not want to alarm Marge, but I was concerned about the possibility of many gruesome things: brain tumor, a stroke, cancer. Encephalitis, a brain infection, could cause behavior like this. A bleed into his brain would be sudden and devastating. Most of these would leave him with catastrophic brain damage.

I thought about him saving teenaged Blake's life—one of the finest ER moments. Desperation welled up. Eric could not go out like this.

I cradled his head and opened his eyes with my fingers. They meandered and then focused on me. He opened his mouth to speak, but no noise came out. He closed his eyes and began snoring.

No! This cannot be happening!

Snoring is a sign of deeply depressed consciousness; he probably had a bleed in his brain. He will die soon.

Where are the paramedics?

Missy burst in. She hugged Marge and took the girls into an adjacent room. She hugged and tried to reassure them.

He opened his eyes and focused on me. He mouthed words and finally said, "What're you doing here?"

"Marge called me. What happened?"

He faded and did not answer.

I heard the ambulance approaching. The lights shone through the windows of the house as they pulled into his driveway.

The paramedics unloaded their stretcher and Missy let them in. I told the story and said that we were both emergency doctors.

They took his blood pressure, pulse, blood sugar, and oxygen levels: all normal. The lead paramedic asked Marge questions.

Eric looked at me and smiled, an altered, flabby smile. I said, "Eric, can you hear me?"

He said, "Yeah" and then slowly winked at me. Not a normal wink, a slow motion wink, but a wink nonetheless. I knew that he could not be joking; he had taken this way too far to be pulling a stunt.

I said, "Do you hurt?"

The lead paramedic was on one knee next to Eric. He abruptly spun toward me and held up his hand, his palm facing me. "It's my turn to ask the questions. You had your turn. We have it under control." He turned back toward Eric.

You have got to be kidding me: a puffed up pufferfish declaring a turf battle in my friend's living room like a kindergartner with a badge and a smidgen of power.

I didn't say anything, but I wanted to karate chop him in the back of the head.

He asked Eric, "Does anything hurt?"

Wow, that was creative. I wonder where you came up with that question?

Eric said, "No." He was slowly looking around, his eyes unfocused. He tried to sit up. "What happened?"

The paramedic said, "We need to get you to a hospital, now. You probably had a stroke."

He said, "No, I'm fine. I'm feeling better." He sat up.

The paramedic said, "We're going to lift you on the stretcher for transport."

"No, I don't think I need to go. I'm all right. Maybe I just drank too much."

Marge said, "Eric, what happened to you? You were totally unconscious."

He said, "I don't know what happened, but I'm fine now."

The paramedic said, "You don't look fine. We need to get you to a hospital as soon as possible."

He said, "I don't want to go."

The paramedics started discussing amongst themselves. Eric turned to me and mouthed, "Help me."

I was becoming convinced that whatever his problem, I could deal with it. He was not going be intubated or need emergency surgery in the next hour. He seemed intoxicated.

I said, "How about this? I'll stay with him and figure this out. If I can't figure out what happened, I'll call you back or take him to the hospital myself."

The paramedic said, "I don't think that's a good idea."

The lead paramedic made a final push to convince Eric to go to the hospital, but he declined. They had him sign forms refusing transport against medical advice and they left.

Marge said with a tremulous voice, "Oh sweetie, I was so worried about you. What happened?" She wrapped her arms around his shoulders and he leaned into her.

I said, "Man, you looked stoned out of your gourd. Did you take any other medicine today?"

He said, "I feel bombed. But no, all I had was a drink or two at dinner. I feel like I've had three pitchers of margaritas. Holy-moly, I'm spinning!"

Marge said, "You seemed blazed. You look like you're on acid or something."

He said defensively, "I swear I haven't taken anything!"

I asked, "Did you take any other medicine today, any cough medicine or whatever?"

"I took Valtrex for a cold sore I was developing. But that shouldn't do anything like this."

"Yeah, that shouldn't make you groggy." I was thinking. We sat silent for a moment.

I said, "Is there any chance something else was in the bottle?"

Marge said, "Maybe that's what happened! I put Ambien in that bottle."

I said, "Really? You put Ambien in the Valtrex bottle? How many pills did you take?"

He smiled knowingly, "Two. I took two."

I burst out laughing. He had taken two Ambien sleeping pills on top of a couple of margaritas. Many ER doctors take sleeping aids to deal with shift work. Ambien and alcohol is a very potent, but harmless, mix.

I laughed, "You took double dose Ambien and washed it down with tequila! Sherlock Holmes ain't got nothing on me!"

Everyone relaxed. I was the only one really laughing, but Marge and Missy smiled. His daughters looked puzzled but relieved.

Eric said, "I'll never live this down. What a lightweight! I have to go lie down; I can hardly keep my eyes open."

I said, "I wouldn't say you are a lightweight. Did you hear what happened to Jeff Palmer?" Jeff was an ER doctor friend.

He chuckled and shook his head, "Yeah, I heard that story."

Marge asked, "What happened?"

I said, "Several of our friends were flying to Hawaii. They were hanging out in the airport sports bar waiting to board. After a few beers, he decided to take an Ambien so he could sleep on the plane. The others told him to wait until he got on the plane, but he took it in the bar. Five minutes later he squirted ketchup on Noah and threw food from his plate. He stumbled over and sat at the table of total strangers. He laughed and talked loudly, acting like a complete jerk. He was almost unable to walk. He was slobbering as he stood in line to get on the plane. Everyone was worried they might not let him board."

Eric said, "On that note, I'm going to bed. Goodnight to all, and to all a good night." He slowly walked up the stairs, both hands tightly gripping the handrails.

◫   ◫   ◫

The next time I saw Eric, I was walking in to begin a shift. He shook his head with an embarrassed grin. I burst out laughing. I asked, "Do you want me to keep your stroke a secret?"

He said, "No, I don't care. That was hilarious. I don't mind being the brunt of the joke." I smiled. It takes a lot of self-confidence to be comfortable not caring what others think.

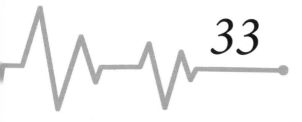

33

I thought about work with a vague malaise. I wondered if I should be seeing more patients per shift. I did not want to be too slow, but I didn't want to rush and make mistakes. I needed to pull my weight. I cared what my new partners thought, maybe too much.

I contemplated a few of the sick people I had discharged: would any of them bounce back? I had a general feeling of disquiet.

I checked my cell phone; there was a message from Noah. He said, "Call me back, no matter what hour. I'm so angry I could kill." Click. The message ended. Noah often left funny messages, but this did not sound like a joke.

I called him back. He said, "I found out who Dr. Judas is. You aren't going to believe this! It's Franklin Trader! He's going to testify against me, the backstabber!"

I felt like I had been hit with the sharp end of a hammer. I said, "What is wrong with him?"

"He's the reason I'm being sued! My lawyer said their case was weak without him! He said the firm wouldn't have taken the case were it not for his willingness to testify! He's their best weapon and our biggest problem! Franklin Traitor!"

"Does he have no decency? I'm so angry I can't see straight."

"I really think that if I saw him on the street, I'd run him over."

"Not if I saw him first."

"I wonder if he knows how this will make him look to the ER community."

"That guy's pathologically twisted. Who knows what he thinks."

"Not only am I an ER doc in the same town, we were in residency together! It defies belief!"

We talked for a few more minutes and made plans to get together later that night. My anger verged on irrationality. I had never been so mad, mad like a madman.

Franklin Trader was threatening Noah's reputation and his finances. He was destroying the happy guy I loved. With three million dollars in debt, Noah would not be able to get a mortgage.

He caused me so much angst during residency; I thought I would never see him again. The emotions of the final year of residency were still raw: Franklin sneaking, and conniving, all the while with a squeaky smile on his face, his teeth sparkling, and his hair just so.

He was back. With a vengeance.

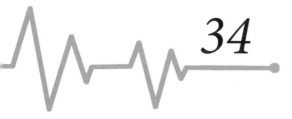

34

I began my shift. I felt grumpy, as my thoughts were littered with Dr. Traitor. I tried to push him out of my mind to concentrate on work.

I asked the partner I was relieving what I could do to help. He transferred care of a patient, a man with depression.

The patient had been in the ER for several days and had been passed from doctor to doctor; half our group had seen him. There are more psychiatric patients in the country than psychiatric hospital beds. Many psychiatric patients cannot hold a job and therefore lack insurance. Psychiatric care loses money for hospitals. Often psychiatric patients spend days in the ER waiting for a bed.

I went to re-evaluate him, working like a psychiatrist, not something I was trained to do. If he was better, maybe I could discharge him with outpatient follow up.

I shook hands with Phillip and his wife, Nhu. He was Caucasian; she was a striking woman of Asian descent, possibly Thai. They appeared healthy and well dressed. He did not smile and barely made eye contact. She smiled, but her onyx eyes betrayed recent tears.

"You haven't been feeling well?"

He spoke in a clipped British accent, "I guess not." He stared straight ahead at the wall. "No, not really."

I sat silently for about ten seconds until it became clear that he was not going to say more.

"Can you tell me how you're feeling?"

He fingered his wire-rimmed glasses. He spoke in a whisper, "Bad."

Nhu spoke up, "Phillip's had a tough year. He's a wonderful father and husband; we've been together for twenty years. He owns a successful company. He's always been a positive, happy person.

"About six months ago he began to withdraw. He didn't want to attend our daughters' school events, a big change. He got angry at things that never bothered him before: at politicians on television, or a neighbor's shoddy mowing. He seemed more and more distant.

"He sat in darkened rooms for hours, then for days on end. He'd cry and not be able to explain what he was crying about.

"I made him an appointment with a psychiatrist a few months ago. He started taking antidepressants. I had to practically drag him to subsequent appointments.

"I tried to get him to snap out of it. I tried to cheer him and convince him how much he had to be happy about. I'd cook his favorite meals and he wouldn't eat them. I'd turn on his favorite music and he'd turn it off. His spark faded."

She quickly wiped away tears. She stopped talking and stared at the wall, her chin quivering.

I looked at Phillip, "Do you feel like you're better or worse than you were a few weeks ago?"

He looked at me with a vacant look, a combination of pain and apathy, like a wounded fawn being toyed with by a lion. "I'm hurting those around me. It'd be better for everyone if I were gone. Nhu can do better."

She submerged her face in her hands and began to weep.

I felt awkward. I wanted to hug her or say something comforting.

His depression seemed profound and wretched. Even worse, it seemed to be caused by nothing. No death, divorce, or loss. If we had a cause, we could deal with it. There was just dark, dirty, black depression, like a coalmine.

I asked, "Have you had thoughts of suicide?"

She wept openly, "That's why we're here. I found him researching guns on the internet."

He said, "I think that's probably the best thing for all. Buy a gun, load the shells, put it in my mouth, pull the trigger, end the pain." I winced involuntarily.

Nhu gasped and began crying uncontrollably. She wilted against her knees and hugged herself as she rocked.

I ached for Nhu. She seemed like a normal suburban soccer mom. They seemed like a family anyone would welcome as friends. I was haunted by the contrast between her beauty and her grinding grief.

I said, "I think you should stay." He continued to stare at the wall as she sobbed, alone.

I awkwardly excused myself. Philip had already been placed on a legal hold. He was being held against his will.

Frequently, family members or the police bring patients like Phillip to the ER. New information has changed the way we think about depression. Depression is related to biochemical changes in the brain and a decrease in serotonin—a brain chemical. Most modern antidepressants are selective serotonin reuptake inhibitors, SSRIs. They increase serotonin.

Of course, depression can be caused by circumstances, such as the death of a loved one, or the death of love. If a negative event causes a worsened mood, there is a measurable decrease in serotonin, a chicken-or-egg phenomenon. Negative events result in depressed moods, decreasing serotonin and driving the mood lower.

Sometimes, serotonin is diminished as a purely biological phenomenon. The person will perceive circumstances negatively.

"My wife is selfish. How did I get stuck with her?" The spouse has not changed, but the perception has, due to biochemical changes in the brain.

Of course, if the wife is treated poorly, she will react; a vicious cycle spins like sharpened blades: cutting, wounding, and destroying.

Under normal circumstances, the patient has the final word on what happens to their bodies. If someone has a heart attack, but decides to leave the ER against medical advice, we will attempt to convince the patient to stay. But if they are deemed competent, they are free to go. The catch-22 is being "deemed competent." One could argue that no one refusing treatment of a heart attack is competent. On the other hand, the weight of societal opinion is: unless a person is intoxicated or mentally deficient, they should be allowed to refuse treatment.

If someone wants to have a DNR status, or Do Not Resuscitate, all they have to do is sign a simple form. Medical professionals will honor their wishes. Often, we spend a lot of effort, and society's money, resuscitating people who are inevitably dying. Performing CPR on a patient with terminal cancer, or a 90-year-old, makes most doctors cringe.

On the other hand, we do not allow people to control their bodies and destinies regarding suicide. The logic is that being suicidal is incongruent with being competent or rational, although the same argument could be made for someone who refuses treatment of a heart attack. If someone says they are suicidal, we hold and treat them against their will, until they are no longer suicidal.

Or until they say they are no longer suicidal.

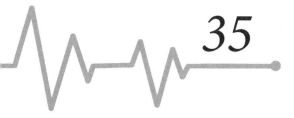

35

I had a mild headache and felt a bit fuzzy from a nap and Benadryl. I gulped bitter coffee to drown the narcosis and to trick my body into thinking it was 8 a.m. instead of 8 p.m. I parked and walked through the parking lot. I noticed a full, yellow-stained, moon.

There is a superstition that the ER is busier, or weirder, when the moon is full. Emergency workers are like athletes: a superstitious bunch. I was not superstitious…at least not until 8 a.m. the following morning.

The events of this bizarre shift made me a believer—sanctified, glorified, and horrified. My new beliefs did not free me, they enslaved me, and I continue to be a fundamentalist slave to the Cult of the Full Moon.

I took over for a partner. He said, "Welcome to the belly of the beast."

I said, "Is there anything I can do to help?"

"Not really, I'm mired knee deep. I have five patients left to finish; I'll be here another three hours. This evening has been a total freak show."

"Maybe you saw all the weirdness and it'll be calm now."

"You wish. Tonight was the first time I've ever seen a beaver bite. The patient found an injured beaver on the side of the road. She picked it up and it bit right through her hand. The teeth came loose in her hand. She came in with two beaver teeth sticking out both sides of her hand.

"My last patient was the straw that broke my back. Come look at her X-ray; she's twenty years old."

The X-ray showed a full sized toothbrush in her stomach. "How did that get there?"

"She was brushing her teeth and accidentally swallowed it."

"She accidentally swallowed a whole toothbrush? Oops, gulp?"

"That's what she said."

"Do you believe her?"

"I don't know why she'd lie."

"I saw something like this at the University; the girl was bulimic. Maybe she was trying to make herself vomit."

"She's thin."

"As they make themselves vomit, they weaken their gag reflexes. So it takes more and more to make them gag. It's the same as a circus performer sticking a sword down his throat."

"I bet that's right. I will talk with her."

I began seeing patients. Later, I was writing on a chart when I heard a shockingly loud walrus-like bellow. It sounded like a trucker's horn blaring behind me. I almost dropped the chart.

A mammoth young man ran into the hall and a security guard hurried away from him. The patient roared again and chased the guard a few steps. He stopped and shook both fists.

A middle-aged woman followed him into the hall and said, "Michael! Come back in here!"

He lumbered back into the room. I asked a nurse, "What's up with that guy?"

She said, "He's autistic. He's been aggressive recently and cut his fist punching a window."

I went to see him. He was the size of an NFL lineman: probably 6'8" and three hundred pounds. He made no eye contact. His mother said, "Michael acts out when he's in a strange environment. The faster you get him out of the ER, the better."

I carefully looked at his hand. I was wary of any quick movements and I was ready to jump back if he swung. The cuts needed suturing. I ordered an X-ray to look for glass.

Patients like Michael are often difficult. Mentally ill or handicapped people are more likely to have problems, and are harder to diagnose due to communication issues. There is a saying in emergency medicine: schizophrenia is not cardiac protective, meaning you cannot blame someone's complaint of chest pain on schizophrenia because schizophrenics have heart attacks just like the rest of us. In Michael's case, I knew what his injuries were, but it was going to be a challenge to get the X-ray and suture his wounds.

I ordered the X-ray and went to see a different patient. A nurse interrupted, "You have to see the patient the ambulance just brought. She's out of control."

I walked toward the room. The screaming patient ran into the hall. She had a huge lac on her forehead with blood streaming over her eyebrows and onto her cheeks. "You can't keep me here! I know my rights! Let me leave!"

I said, "Ma'am, please go back to your room."

"Who made you king? I want to talk to my lawyer!"

Two security guys escorted her to her room as she screamed and threatened. The paramedic said, "She's drunker than Cooter Brown. Her 7-year-old son called the ambulance because she was so drunk she fell and cut her head. She had a seizure en route to the hospital that lasted about two minutes. She says she's a nurse."

I walked into the room. She shrieked, "I'm leaving! I have rights!"

I said, "You should stay until we sort this out. You have a significant cut on your face. That will leave a horrible scar if we don't suture it."

"I don't care about a scar. This is not right. You can't take me out of my house against my will." She thrust her cell phone at me. "Please call my lawyer. His name is Drew Schmertz."

I ignored her phone. "O.K., let's talk about why you're here. What happened?"

"Why should I tell you? It's none of your business. I didn't ask to be brought here!"

Behind the patient, a nurse was going through the patient's belongings. She raised her brow and held up the patient's ID badge. The patient was an ER nurse at another major hospital in town.

I groaned. The fact that she was an ER nurse made this much more complex. I had to be very careful with her in an adversarial role. She would know how to complain. She knew what to say to cause trouble. No matter what I did, she could make me pay.

Sometimes taking care of physicians and nurses is difficult as they have their own ideas. Of course, all patients should be involved in their care, but most don't debate every order. A drunken health care professional would be problematic.

I heard a sea lion bellow in the hall, and I startled a second time. I heard shouting and running. I scrambled out. Michael was running toward the exit and the security guards and nurses wisely stepped out of his way to allow him free exit. He barreled toward the double sliding glass doors of the ambulance entrance. Each door was about ten by ten feet. He slowed in front of the doors momentarily. The doors didn't open. He charged.

He hit the door with his full weight and it shattered with a low boom. The safety glass rained prismatic cubes all over Michael and the floor. The force of the blow knocked him staggering backwards. Several security guards and nurses tried to restrain him; he dropped to one knee.

He fought mightily, King Kong against the world. I rushed up and felt glass grind and pop. I clutched a tree-trunk leg. He thrashed about like the King of Kong restrained by cables, swatting at helicopters.

Often during a takedown of a combative patient, the staff will smirk or roll their eyes. Not this time, we were holding on for dear life and praying he wouldn't overpower the entire gaggle of us.

A nurse stabbed him with a sedative injection. Before the medicine had time to work, he suddenly stopped fighting and lay passively. We strapped him to a gurney and rolled him to his room. I surveyed his injuries and found several new cuts that needed suturing. I was originally worried about sewing up his hand. Now, I had his hand, his back, his shoulder, his scalp, his temper, his enormousness. My simple plan for Michael got complicated.

Quagmire.

His mother said, "He will not tolerate the restraints. If he's tied down for more than a few minutes, he'll fight. Once he starts fighting, he won't stop. There's no way you'll be able to sew his cuts." I asked the nurse to remove his restraints.

I spoke with his mother outside the room, "I'm going to order X-rays of his deeper cuts to look for glass. What's the best way to proceed with suturing?"

"The calmer the environment, the calmer he'll be. We can turn on the TV and I'll sit quietly. Just walk in softly and start working. If you ignore him, hopefully he'll ignore you."

"Do you think he might get violent?"

"It's possible. Usually, he gives a warning before he hits."

"Usually?" I did not like the sound of that.

"I'll watch. If I say 'Doctor,' jump up as fast as you can and run out."

Jump up and run out? I might be holding a needle and syringe, looking down at the wound, when King Kong's fist—the size of my face—smashes me. He might knock me into the wound and into the sharp scissors, tweezers, and needles. He might strike repeatedly.

"OK. I'll be back after I see his X-rays." I felt uneasy, to say the least.

I went to speak with the intoxicated nurse. She ranted, cussed, and raved some more, "I'm going to sue. I hope you have a good lawyer, because I do!"

I said, "Your son called the ambulance because you're so drunk you fell. You cut your head and had a seizure. You aren't competent to refuse care. You have to stay until we've done a CAT scan of your head, and you're more sober."

"This isn't fair! I'm not drunk! I haven't had much to drink!" Each slurred word blew aerosolized Jim Beam toward my face. My hair wilted.

I saw a few more patients. I saw a 70-year-old woman who was confused. Her husband said, "We've been here over two hours and nothing's been done! What's going on? Should we go to a different ER? What's wrong with you people?"

I said, "I'm sorry, sir. This is an incredibly busy night and we're trying as hard as we can. We normally have about half as many patients."

I turned to the patient, "What's bothering you today? Why are you here?"

She said, "I don't know why I'm here, and you need to quit being rude."

Her husband said, "We didn't come to be treated like second class citizens!"

"I'm sorry. I don't mean to be rude. She's been confused?"

"I've already told the story to three people! Didn't you read her chart?"

"I'm sorry this is frustrating. I read she's been confused. Can you tell me more? The more info I have, the more we can help."

He softened a bit and said she had been increasingly confused over a few days. I ordered a CAT scan of her brain, blood tests, a chest X-ray, and a urine test. I hurried to see another patient.

Michael's X-rays came back. I didn't see any glass in the wounds. I took a deep breath. I dreaded returning to his room. His hands were big. He was strong. He had a history of violence, and plenty of reasons to be angry.

A few minutes later, I walked in and sat next to him. His mother had calmed him and he was watching television. He stared at the TV while I prepared quietly. I warily watched for any sudden movements or signs of agitation. I held my breath as I prepared to inject lidocaine into his skin with a long needle. The needle paused above his skin, trembling.

I pushed it in.

He winced but didn't react otherwise. I slowly exhaled. I sutured in silence for about twenty minutes.

I discussed his discharge plan with his mother and arranged his discharge. She thought he would try to run again if brought into the main ER. Security placed his arms and legs in soft restraints; he seemed sedated from the tranquilizer. She left the ER to get her van. We rolled him into the parking lot. His mother called from the van, "Michael. I'm over here."

They removed all four restraints at once and he bolted upright, ran full speed to the car, and jumped in with a single bound.

I returned to the ER and a nurse told me the confused elderly woman had dangerously low blood sugar. I ordered IV glucose and food. All of her other tests came back normal.

I spoke with her husband. "She had very low blood sugar and that's why she's confused. I'm not sure why her sugar has been low but she needs admission to monitor her sugar and complete her workup."

He agreed. He was pleasant and shook my hand. He went home at 2 a.m.

The plastered nurse's CT scan was normal. She muttered and cursed the entire time I sutured her wounds. Her seizure was probably due to the blow to her head from her fall. With a negative CT, she was safe to go home. I discharged her.

I was done seeing patients and sat to dictate charts. The morning doctor would arrive soon. I was exhausted, beat down. Night shifts are hard enough when work flows smoothly. I rubbed my eyes. I rifled through the tall stack of charts, procrastinating. I tried to concentrate.

A nurse called my portable phone, "The confused woman says she wants to leave. She's acting kooky and keeps trying to get out of bed. I rechecked her blood sugar and it's normal."

I went to speak with the patient. She was trying to climb out of the bed and a nurse attempted to stop her.

She said, "You people are holding me hostage. I'm going to escape!"

"What's wrong? Why do you want to leave?"

"This is a prison camp. I know you torture people." She began screaming loud enough for most of the ER to hear, "Help! I'm being kidnapped! Please, someone help me! Help!"

A confused grandma, a snockered nurse, a gigantic Michael, and a pitiful ER doctor all agreed on one thing: let's fly this coop. Let's get the heck out of Dodge. This place is cursed.

I did not care anymore. I had to leave. I had to. I was beyond wit's end. I grabbed her hand, pulled her out of bed, and sprinted through the shattered ambulance bay door, crunching glass underfoot and holding hands as we escaped into the night. She ran fast for a grandma. I heard nurses yelling but I didn't look back. In the parking lot, she hugged me tight, kissed my cheek, and we jumped into my car, like Bonnie and Clyde.

I revved the engine and spun the stereo volume to eleven, cranking AC/DC. Blue smoke floated from my tires as I did donuts in the parking lot. She drained a Bud, sparked a Marlboro, and took a hard drag. She put on my sunglasses, smiled calmly, and said, "Right on, bro!"

In my rearview mirror, I saw a crowd of astonished nurses as I fishtailed out of the parking lot, on the way to Vegas casinos and Mexican nightclubs.

I wished. I wished, wished, wished.

I snapped out of my fantasies, staring at her scream, "Help! Police!" I could see her tonsils.

I said, "O.K. I will help you. I'm here to make sure you aren't tortured."

"Thank you, doctor. Keep those evil people away." She seemed to think we were on the same team.

I called her husband. I hoped he could talk some sense into her. I told him the situation and handed the phone to his wife. I left the room and limped back to my stack of dictations.

About 30 minutes later, the nurse found me. She said, "Her husband's here to take her home! He's refusing the admission. The transport guy was pushing her wheelchair, taking her to her room upstairs. As he was leaving the ER, the husband ran up and said, 'You aren't taking her anywhere!' He grabbed the wheelchair and rolled her toward the exit. Will you come talk with him?"

I walked up. He was facing me, standing behind the wheelchair. He yelled, "Get out of my way! I'm taking her out of this place!

You people are demented!" He looked at me, "And you, sir, will be hearing from my lawyer!"

I thought, maybe you and Nurse Slurry can get a two-for-one deal on a lawyer.

I said, "I'm sorry you're upset, but she really needs to be admitted. Her blood sugar was dangerously low. If her sugar drops again, it could cause permanent brain damage or even kill her."

He wagged his finger at me, "I don't trust a single one of you. Now get out of my way or I will run you over." He lowered his head, and pushed the wheelchair toward me like he was going to plow me under. I stood my ground and he fortunately stopped. I was pleased to avoid a collision between the metal wheelchair and my shins. His face twisted furiously and he spewed venom.

I pled with him for 10 minutes to no avail. He was competent and was next of kin. He signed forms refusing care. He wheeled his wife into the dark parking lot.

I was slack jawed. He was doing what I wanted to do, escape.

But the logical side of me worried. Sometimes we cautiously admit people to the hospital that might be fine to go home. She was not one of those patients. She really needed to be hospitalized. The brain will fry in short order when the blood sugar is too low. I wondered if she were already brain damaged from previous episodes of low blood sugar.

Later, I called her husband on the phone. He said, "She's fine. She's asleep. We both were asleep before you called!"

"She could have very low blood sugar. Will you bring her back tomorrow morning?"

"No."

"At least check her blood sugar every two hours and bring her back if it's below sixty."

He grunted noncommittally and hung up.

I began dictating. My throat was sore and my brain was also. The dictations were painful.

A nurse rushed up, "Brent, we have a terrible nosebleed in here. It can't wait until the morning doc gets here. He's bleeding like a hydrant. He's on blood thinners."

I walked to the patient's room. He was an elderly man with eyes of fear. Blood covered his face like a heinous beard, clots dangling from his chin. I grabbed gloves and a suction catheter.

I had never believed the myth of the Full Moon. It seemed like a bunch of superstitious mumbo-jumbo.

I believe. Believe me, I'm a believer. I was immersed in the lake of fire and brimstone, baptism by fire. I was baptized against my will. My soul was sold to the spirits of the night. The die was cast and I became a fearful man, battered by powers beyond my understanding. I needed candles, a skull, and a chicken for a blood sacrifice to pacify the demon voodoo priests of the Cult of the Full Moon.

I looked at my watch: two more hours until the Moon vanishes and the sun arrives. I ached to escape the menace of the capricious power of the lidless eye, the glaring Moon.

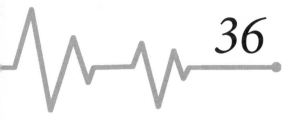

36

I drove back to Portland after attempting to ski. A powerful Pacific storm had blown in; the wind was so strong, the lifts never ran. I drove two hours and turned around, not exactly the outing I had hoped for. The storm caused accidents on the highway and I spent most of the day sitting in the car. I was stressed I might be late for my evening shift.

The roads finally opened up and the smell of the fir-scented forest faded as strip malls and asphalt replaced trees and ski trails. The two-lane road changed to four, to eight. Skyscrapers graffitied the sky and replaced the strip malls of the suburbs. The speed and the volume of the motorized traffic grew exponentially the closer I got to the city. Motorcycles and compact cars navigated perilously between SUVs and trucks—like a Serengeti migration: monkeys and gazelles zigging and zagging under the feet of stampeding elephants. The autos drove faster and closer as more lanes were added to the chaos.

We were like small stars being pulled into the black hole, a vortex from which there was no escape.

I pondered the recent drama. Sometimes I felt like my life was speeding toward a destructive force. Little bits and pieces were falling off as I screamed toward the black hole.

A black hole creates a gravitational pull inward, a crushing under your own weight. My life was crushing under its heaviness. As I added layer upon layer, I had complicated my life, a burdensome array of responsibilities, expectations, and possessions—carrying them through life like a chain over my back.

If you think you have a lot; you think you have a lot to lose.

I dwelled on Noah's trial too much, and my distaste for Franklin grew. I had never loathed anyone before; I probably couldn't name more than three people I did not like. I had to get my anger in check.

I felt gun shy at work. Every patient seemed like an adversary, someone who might sue: another opportunity for mistake or error.

Maybe we are like the Twin Towers, a complex structure that only needs one problem, a lawsuit—flown by a crazed pilot to bring the entire thing down under its own weight: crashing, splintering, and destroying everything around it in a smoldering heap. I worried about Noah's relationships.

I hated feeling this way. I knew it was wrong. I shouldn't let Franklin under my skin. My chances of being sued had not increased because Noah had been sued. It was ludicrous, but I still felt that way.

I parked at the hospital and took a deep breath. I went inside to start my shift. The first patient was a small, young man who had been battered by his very large, and very drunk, girlfriend. The nurse snickered, "A wimp and a blimp." I felt awkward at the joke as his girlfriend had knocked him down and broken his ankle in three places.

I was thankful the shift was slow. I saw a pregnant patient with bleeding and awaited her ultrasound results. I admitted a middle-aged man with a blood clot in his lung.

I dreaded speaking with the woman who claimed kidney stones and wanted narcotics. I checked her computerized medical records; she had been in the ER about thirty times in the past year for a variety of pain-related complaints. Several times she had blood in her urine but the CAT scans for kidney stones had been negative. The previous doctor who had seen her in the ER recommended no more narcotics. I needed to go along with the plan, but I hated conflict, especially with patients.

I entered her room. "Dr. Jones talked with you the last time you were here about the problems with narcotics."

She said, "My back's killing me. I haven't been able to sleep. I'm miserable."

"It's not healthy to take narcotics chronically. Addictive medicines create tolerance. For long-term problems, narcotics aren't the answer."

"It's not a long-term problem. I can't help that I have kidney stones."

"Over the past year, you've been in the ER multiple times for different things. You've received many prescriptions for narcotics. Every time a CAT scan has been done for kidney stones, it's been negative."

"I don't want to be on pain meds long term. I just need something this week. I won't ask again; I have to sleep."

I really wanted to prescribe narcotics and keep moving. That would be much easier and quicker. Maybe she did really have pain.

I thought about my good friend, Karen. We had gone to high school and college together. We dated, but were mostly close friends, although I always had a bit of a crush on her. She was beautiful and popular with a charming, funny personality. She was a cheerleader and on the Homecoming Court.

She partied in high school and college, but nothing out of the ordinary. Shortly after I finished residency, one bright, blue day turned into a dark, blue day when I heard the news—Karen was dead. She died from complications related to a narcotic pill addiction.

I called her sister. She said Karen had gotten most of her narcotics from ER doctors. She said, "Karen could charm anyone, and she always got what she wanted."

The demons had taken another victim: a beautiful, special person who was exceptional in every way. They had stolen from the angels, and had stolen from me.

I said, "I'd like to try something non-narcotic for your pain. Have you tried ibuprofen or Tylenol?"

"Are you saying I'm a drug addict? There's blood in my urine! Why should that other doctor be in charge of my treatment?"

I said, "Let me look you over again." I examined her back and then gripped her left hand. When I squeezed her fingertips, a drop of blood welled up from her ring finger. Her eyes widened—busted!

I said, "I'm going to put your chart up for discharge."

I walked out of the room. I began filling out her discharge papers. Her nurse asked, "How did it go with the woman in room seven?"

"She put up a good fight, until I squeezed her hand where she'd pricked her finger to put blood in her urine sample. She looked like a deer in the high beams."

The nurse laughed.

The overhead speaker squawked loudly, "Code Blue, Eastern Parking Garage. Code Blue, Eastern Parking Garage." I was the doctor assigned for codes. Sometimes codes are called for someone fainting or being too weak to walk. A true Code Blue is someone who is not breathing or has no pulse. But at Brookwood, and I suspect most hospitals, it is often called for much less than that.

If it is in the ICU or the cardiac ward, it is likely to be a real Code Blue. If it is in the cafeteria or parking garage, chances are grandma slipped on a banana peel. Of course, I couldn't assume, but that was what I expected as I ran toward the exit of the ER.

Two nurses and a tech with a rolling stretcher were running toward the same exit. We charged into the street in front of the hospital that led to the parking garage. I took the lead.

As I rounded a corner, I saw a crowd of people in front of the five-story parking garage. There were about twenty people standing in a loose circle in the street. I said loudly, "Excuse us. Dr. Russell from the ER." We broke through the crowd.

I was not prepared for what we saw.

There was an internal medicine resident doing chest compressions on a bloody figure. The resident's crisp white blouse was splattered with crimson drops. Blood bubbled out of the patient's mouth and ears with each chest compression. The resident had a dazed, horribly vacant look.

"What happened?" I asked.

She said softy, "He jumped."

There was a fine spray of maroon on her glasses and blood flecks on her cheeks.

I dropped to my knees and said, "Stop CPR." I felt for a pulse. Nothing.

I touched the back of the head and felt his skull, broken fragments held together by skin and matted hair.

My finger poked through; I felt his brain.

"Let's put him on the stretcher and go to the ER." I knew he was dead, but wanted to remove him from the scene.

We heaved him onto the gurney. I said, "To the ER." We began moving away. I saw a face in the crowd. It was a young woman with an unholy look of grief on her face.

I froze.

A look of misery. A look of agony. I stared at the most anguished eyes I had ever seen, and I had seen those very eyes before. Our eyes connected and her onyx eyes poured darkness into mine.

Nhu, Phillip's wife.

I tore myself away from the flow of infinite sorrow.

I was confused as we rushed toward the ER. What happened?

Wasn't Phillip a patient on the psychiatric ward? Why was he on top of the parking garage?

When we arrived in the ER, we put Phillip on a cardiac monitor. Flatline.

He was declared dead less than one minute after arriving in the ER. I noticed his hands were uninjured; he had not put out his hands when he struck the ground. He had been dead the moment he hit the pavement.

I waited a few minutes before walking out of the ER to talk with Nhu. I did not want her to think we had done nothing for him, even though there was nothing to do. It felt odd to rush to the ER and then walk out two minutes later.

I dreaded speaking with her. I would rather have seen a million narcotic drug seekers than face her. I was not sure I could endure her eyes again.

I slowly walked to the family conference room. Nhu was alone.

I said, "I met you a few weeks ago in the ER. I'm so sorry. Phillip is dead."

I could tell she already knew; she was not crying. She looked like a prisoner of war, drained of her humanity. She stared at the ground.

She said, "I can't believe it. I thought he was getting better. I can't..." She paused and stared, then continued, "He told his psychiatrist he was no longer suicidal. They let him come home for several hours today and he was supposed to return to the hospital to spend the night.

"He came home and hugged the girls. He didn't smile but he didn't cry. We had a 'Welcome Home Daddy' poster. We went for a long walk.

"When we returned to the hospital and stepped in the elevator, I pushed the button to the seventh floor. Just as the doors were closing, he bolted. The doors closed and I had to ride all the way to the seventh floor. I was hysterical.

"When I got back to the ground floor, I ran looking for him. I had no idea what he was doing, but I knew it wasn't good. I ran around outside helplessly—panicking, hoping, hunting. I saw a crowd gathering in the street.

"As I ran up, I asked a woman walking away from the scene what had happened. She told me that a man had jumped from the parking garage."

She paused. She raised her coal eyes.

"I entered the circle and saw a young woman trying to revive him. I turned around and stood outside the crowd. I couldn't watch.

"I looked up and realized that he could see the parking garage from his hospital room window. He'd jumped off the parking garage onto the one place there was pavement; there's grass on three sides. He'd planned the jump from his hospital bed."

◫ ◫ ◫

I arrived home late after seeing Phillip. I trudged up the front steps—I needed to scream, I needed to be silent, I needed company, I needed solitude, I wanted to sleep, I was frightened of nightmares.

I wanted to stand on my head and let the darkness drain out like ink: reversing today, reversing everything.

Missy was still awake, sitting on the couch with a novel. She smiled warmly. I forced a smile and kissed her. She asked, "How was your day?"

I swallowed, "Fine." I paused, "Yours?"

She said, "All's well with the second graders. They never cease to make me laugh." She went on to tell me a story from her day at school.

I nodded. She asked if I wanted pancakes for breakfast. I stared blankly at a *Newsweek*.

Nhu stared back.

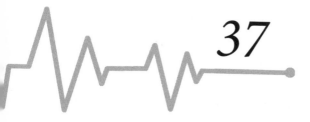

37

A week later, I left a shift at Brookwood and headed toward the Wallowa mountain range in Eastern Oregon. I was meeting my two brothers for a backcountry ski trip.

I was looking forward to the trip. The Wallowas are as spectacular as anything in the U.S., but few people visit. If you came up with a value that took the beauty of an area and divided it by the number of visitors per year, the Wallowas would score high.

The Wallowas are similar to Yosemite: sheer cliffs of white granite, shockingly blue lakes, unspoiled forests, and cascading waterfalls. In the winter, the mountains look like the Alps.

I pulled onto the highway and set the cruise control. I was glad to see Portland in my rear view mirror.

I was looking forward to getting away: my last hurrah before Noah's trial. I needed a break from everything: Franklin, work, lawsuits, suicides. I couldn't get Nhu's pitch-dark eyes out of my mind.

I still had not told Missy about Phillip and Nhu. It was not breakfast conversation to discuss fatherless daughters holding a "Welcome Home Daddy" poster. I couldn't talk about blood oozing from his ears while Missy brushed her teeth.

I have seen many attempted suicides in my years as a doctor. Most people who succeed—gunshots or jumping from high places—never end up in the ER; the paramedics declare them dead at the scene.

Our primary human instinct is survival. Our biology, our intellect, our soul, and our spirit all scream, "Survive! Live!" That intolerable sadness and misery will overwhelm such a primal instinct is astonishing.

Suicide is nonexistent in many poor parts of the world; people are too busy trying to survive. They don't have time to dwell on their grief or lack of contentment.

I drove along and my mind drifted into dreary territory. I thought of suicides I had seen.

One patient tried to commit suicide by cutting his own throat with a razor blade. He cut his trachea in half, but missed his jugular and carotids. He came into the ER with a gaping hole in his neck.

I was a med student. The ER doctor slid the endotracheal tube into the patient's trachea through his neck, instead of his mouth. The patient lived; I wondered if he was grateful or if he hated the doctor.

Another patient, Sandra, had been depressed for as long as she could remember. She was separated from her husband. She worked as a real estate agent, but lost her job due to alcoholism. She had been drinking heavily and feeling worse each day. Her alcoholism made her almost homeless; she had been living on a friend's couch prior to coming to the ER.

Sandra came to the ER and said she was suicidal. After about twenty-four hours in the ER at Brookwood, a nurse went to check on her. She was hanging by a bathrobe tie from a cabinet. She had hooked the tie onto the top of the cabinet and tied the other end around her neck.

Her face was mottled and purple, her eyes bulging and lifeless, like twin pool balls. Her bloated tongue parted her lips like a cancer invading a healthy organ. They cut her down and resuscitated her.

She was barely alive. Her pupils did not react; not a soul in the room thought she had a chance to be a normal person. Usually if a patient's pupils are fixed and do not react to light, they are brain dead. If she lived, the most likely outcome was a permanent vegetative state, kept alive with feeding tubes, a fate worse than death.

She spent three weeks in the ICU where she made a remarkable physical recovery. She then went to the psychiatric ward. The psychiatrist thought she was a hopeless case, an alcoholic who would not take responsibility for her choices. He had known her from previous admissions where she blamed others for her problems and was not interested in changing.

He was astonished to find she was engaged in the counseling sessions; she seemed like a new woman. Some thought the hanging was like electroshock therapy, resetting her brain. Others thought she hit bottom and bounced very high.

Several weeks later she came to the ER and asked for the nurse, Ann, who had cut her down. Sandra was well dressed and personable. She thanked Ann. Ann sent an email to the entire ER staff about how Sandra and her recovery had given Ann a new respect and love for her job.

Another time, I took a call from an excited paramedic who said, "I'm calling to see if I should take this patient to the trauma hospital or bring him to your ER. He's an inmate at the county jail and he hanged himself with a toothbrush!"

I asked, "He hanged himself with a toothbrush?"

"Yes, can we bring him there?"

I said "Sure." I wondered how he could hang himself with a toothbrush.

When he arrived the patient had blood covering his face and a toothbrush sticking out of his nose. The paramedics had intubated him. He had not hanged himself, but had sharpened his toothbrush, stuck it in his nose, and struck it with the base of his palm. The toothbrush had broken through a thin part of the skull, where the olfactory nerves enter the brain.

His CAT scan showed air throughout the brain. The neurosurgeon said he had no chance of survival. We did not try to keep him alive; he died in the ER.

The most disturbing case was a middle-aged man who shot himself in the temple. The bullet went anterior to the brain, straight through the eye sockets. The bullet shattered both of his eyeballs, but missed his brain.

He came into the ER at the University, conscious and talking, with eyeball shards protruding from his eyelids; it looked like broken egg shells sticking out of his sockets. He said, "Just let me die."

I intubated him in the ER. About twelve hours later, I went to see how he was doing in the ICU.

He was unconscious and on a ventilator. His brain had begun to swell. His adult son arrived.

His son walked in the room and watched his father from a few feet away. He wiped away tears and said, "Dad, you probably cannot hear me but if you can, I want to tell you something before you die."

I felt uneasy to witness such an intimate moment. I was sure that his son was going to pour out loving emotion or regret.

He said loudly, "I hate you! I hope you rot in hell!"

He stormed out, cursing.

Over the next few days the patient's brain swelled; his brain stuck out of his shattered eye sockets, like a fly's bulging gray eyes. The son did not want to turn off the ventilator. He said, "Keep that man alive so he suffers as long as possible."

Often family members want to keep someone alive against all odds, hoping for a miracle. The son desired an evil miracle. He prayed a twisted prayer to the Prince of Darkness for maximum suffering, that the Angel of Death would take a piece each day leaving the father in tormented limbo—a blinded suffering zombie.

The ethics committee of the hospital was consulted and they recommended a withdrawal of life support. The man died a few hours after the vent was turned off.

I blinked my eyes to rid my thoughts of the macabre. I do not like thinking such depressing thoughts. I exited on I-84 and headed into the Columbia Gorge.

I shook my head: Snap out of it, Brent. Stop thinking fetid thoughts. The purpose of this trip is to get away from it all, not foul my mind with images of human carnage.

I vowed to think only cheerful thoughts for the weekend: no thinking about the trial and Dr. Traitor, no thinking about gaping tracheas, brain-covered toothbrushes, or a bitter son cursing his blind father.

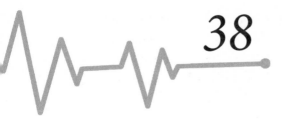

38

The fire was everywhere. Smoke filled the room. The ceiling was on fire and hot timbers fell on the bed. I needed to get up, run, and jump out a window, but I was too sleepy to get out of bed. The fire alarm was ringing. Ringing. Ringing. I needed to get up but the pillow was so soft. Ringing. Ringing.

I opened my eyes and realized the phone was ringing, and my room was cool and dark. I rolled over to answer. "Hello."

Noah said, "Were you asleep?"

"Yeah. I worked late last night. Today's the day, huh?"

"I'm on my way to the gallows. My tie feels like a noose."

"How do you feel?"

"Like sticking a sharpened toothbrush into my brain."

"This, too, shall pass. Call me tonight and fill me in."

⊞   ⊞   ⊞

A few minutes later Noah was listening to the lawyer for the plaintiff. "My client, Jerome Bristol, was severely injured by the combined malpractice of Bluefield Hospital, Health First Ambulances, the cardiologist, Dr. Al Heller, and the emergency physician, Dr. Noah Jackson.

"My client was in excellent heath on October sixteenth when he suffered a major heart attack. He's the vice president of a major bank, a father of two sons, and a devoted husband of twenty-six years. He was an avid golfer and fisherman.

"After the substandard treatment he received that fateful day, he's now unable to work a full week. He is unable to do most of the things he used to do, including playing golf or taking an evening stroll.

"We will show that the negligence of the physicians involved in his care injured him in a way that his life has been irreparably injured. His previous existence is a faraway dream. We are asking the jury to consider his loss of wages as well as pain and suffering caused by a life crippled and shortened by the mistreatment of others.

"Bluefield hospital was negligent in several ways. One, they only had one cardiac cath unit when it is clearly possible for more than one person to have a heart attack on any given day. Dr. Noah Jackson was clearly overwhelmed by this case and grossly mismanaged my client's treatment with substandard and sloppy work."

He droned on about how the ambulance company was negligent and how the cardiologist had chosen poorly. Noah was no longer able to concentrate as the insults stung his ears. The public torment was nothing he had ever experienced. He was used to award ceremonies, graduations, smiling audiences, and grateful patients—not scorn and humiliation.

Noah's lawyer began with his opening remarks. "We are all saddened by what happened to Mr. Bristol. None of us would wish this.

"We plan to show that our client, Dr. Jackson, performed above the standard of care in this very difficult case. His patient, Mr. Bristol, would be dead if he'd not been shocked back to life by Dr. Jackson. Dr. Jackson did not cause the original problem in Mr. Bristol's heart and did his best to save Mr. Bristol from further injury. Dr. Jackson performed several life saving interventions with his medical treatment.

"Unfortunately, there were two heart attacks at Bluefield Hospital at the same time. The last time that happened was four years ago. If Bluefield had a second full-time cath team on call it would cost over one million dollars a year. That is not the standard of care and would be an incredible waste of limited heath care resources. There are no hospitals in our state that have two cath teams. None. Not the University, not Brookwood, none.

"We plan to show that, while it's a tragedy when anyone is injured, Mr. Bristol should take responsibility for his heath. He was a heavy smoker and had not seen his doctor in years. He had untreated high blood pressure and high cholesterol. He had been having chest pains for over a week when he finally called the ambulance. To mistreat your body and then sue the well-meaning heath care providers when they are unable to perfectly heal you is misguided. It might strike some as thankless or greedy."

They took a break for lunch. Noah's lawyer said it was going about as he had expected. Reggie said, "You looked angry, Noah. Don't get angry, or at least try not to appear angry. Juries don't like angry doctors."

Noah asked, "What do you think the chances are that we will win?"

Reggie said, "Same as before, less than fifty percent."

Noah sat by himself in a sterile conference room wearing a suit. He sat at a metal table with a peeling wood laminate, on a hard folding chair. He slowly chewed a peanut butter and jelly sandwich.

▣　▣　▣

After the break, Franklin Trader took the stand. He looked distinguished and handsome in a tailor made dark suit. His face was tan and his teeth were unnaturally white. His lawyer asked, "Dr. Trader, are you a board certified Emergency Medicine Physician?"

He replied, "Yes, I am."

"And where do you work?"

"I'm a full-time emergency physician at St Paul's Hospital."

"Do you know Dr. Jackson?"

"With full disclosure, I'd like to say that I am a friend and colleague of Dr. Noah Jackson. We were in residency together and I've always gotten along well with him. It pains me to testify in this case, but my fond feelings for him should be put aside for justice."

"Do you think the emergency care given by Dr. Jackson met the minimum standard of care?"

"No, I do not."

"What would you have done differently?"

"This patient clearly should have been given a clot busting drug as soon as it became apparent the cath lab at Bluefield was unavailable. This is a clearly stated principle in Emergency Medicine textbooks.

"Dr. Jackson did not ask Mr. Bristol what his wishes were. If I had seen Mr. Bristol as a patient, I would have explained the situation and gotten his input, instead of paternalistically playing God."

His lawyer continued, "Dr. Trader, what textbooks are you referring to?"

"The most respected textbook is Principles of Emergency Medicine, originally authored by Dr. Goldfrank. As you can see from page one hundred sixteen, Goldfrank's book clearly shows a flowchart regarding management of heart attacks." He took a laser pointer and shone a red dot onto the blown up page out of the textbook. "Right at this juncture it says that if an EKG shows a heart attack, cardiac cath or a clot busting medicine should be given immediately. Nowhere does it say that long delays are justified."

Noah's lawyer stood to cross-examine. His job was not to argue medicine with a doctor. He would try to soften him up for the eventual damage that, hopefully, Dr. Hans Maier could inflict on him.

"Dr. Trader, where do you work now?"

"I work at St. Paul's."

"Dr. Trader, you said you would've discussed clot busting medicines versus catheterization with Mr. Bristol, correct?"

"Yes. Medical professionals no longer interact with patients in a paternalistic, doctor-knows-best way. A thoughtful doctor will present options to the patient and allow the patient to participate in decisions made."

"I see. What would you have told Mr. Bristol?"

"I would've told him that he could wait to have cardiac catheterization at another hospital or receive a clot busting medicine. I would've recommended a clot busting medicine."

"That's what you would have said?"

"Yes, that's what I would've recommended."

"So, how is this any less paternalistic than what Dr. Jackson did? Is a banker going to tell you he'd rather have a different treatment, other than what the doctor recommends?"

"He should still know the options."

"Have you ever had a patient do something other than what you recommend for treatment of a heart attack?"

"Yes, in fact I have. I had a fellow physician as a patient and he refused open heart surgery."

"A fellow physician? Is that the same as a banker?"

"No, it's not. I'm not here to play gotcha with you. The point I'm trying to make is that Dr. Jackson did the wrong thing and injured Mr. Bristol."

Reggie asked, "Dr. Jackson had a cardiologist in the ER with him as these decisions were made. They decided together that CB wasn't worth the risk. Would you have overridden a heart specialist's advice?"

"Yes, I would have. I would've done what I thought was right rather than commit malpractice."

MIRACLES and MAYHEM in the ER

"Really? What about the fact that the EKG done at the decision point showed that he no longer met criteria for CB?"

Franklin answered, "Do you see anything on this flowchart that says anything about a second EKG? That's a maneuver that doesn't accomplish anything. It's quite silly actually."

Reggie finished, "You had two points. One was that you would have allowed Mr. Bristol to choose his treatment. The jury understands that you cannot explain all of the risks and benefits of such a complex situation to allow a truly informed choice. You also told us that you would recommend a certain course of treatment.

"We are left with your argument that Dr. Jackson should've given a clot busting medicine and overridden the cardiologist. We'll discuss that point later. Thank you, your honor."

The lawsuit went on and on. There were multiple lawyers involved as the lawsuit involved four defendants, the cardiologist, the ambulance company, the hospital and Noah.

Their second doctor, Dr. Dorcas, took the stand. He worked in an urgent care clinic in Northern California.

He gave his testimony: basically the same thing that Franklin had already said. Reggie got up to cross-examine.

"Dr. Dorcas, please tell us where you work and your professional credentials."

"At Redding Urgent Care. I'm a board certified Internal Medicine Doctor."

"Urgent Care. Isn't that for minor injuries and illnesses?"

"We see all types of patients."

"How many heart attacks have you treated in the past three years?"

"Several."

"That you treated. Not someone who came in with chest pain and you called an ambulance to transfer to the local ER while you sat around sweating and doing nothing. How many have you treated?"

"Urgent Care isn't set up to treat serious emergencies like that. We don't have the equipment or the support staff."

"So the answer is zero, correct?"

"Yes, but I know about treatment of myocardial infarctions."

"I did not ask what you know. How many cases have you testified in during the past five years?"

"A few."

"That's not a satisfactory answer. How many?"

"I don't see what that has to do with anything."

"The answer is thirty-five. How many times have you testified that the doctor being sued did not commit malpractice?"

"I'm not sure."

"Let me refresh your memory. The answer is, let's see here." He looked down at his notes dramatically, "It appears the answer is again: zero. Do you care to contradict this?"

"No."

"The defense rests, your honor."

Mr. Bristol's lawyer stood and asked Dr. Dorcas what he thought of Franklin's testimony. Dr. Dorcas delivered a devastating blow to the defense.

"As Dr. Trader showed earlier, here's the flowchart from the authoritative text in Emergency Medicine, from the chapter on how to manage heart attacks. Right here at this branch point, it clearly states that a heart attack should be treated with cardiac cath or clot busters immediately.

"Immediately.

"Why did Dr. Jackson dither while Mr. Bristol's reversible heart problem worsened to the point of irreversibility? Why didn't he learn this most basic point during his residency? Dr. Trader, who was a colleague of Dr. Jackson's during residency, feels that he committed malpractice. His care was substandard.

"Dr. Trader must feel very strongly about this to bravely testify against a wayward colleague, when most medical professionals would turn a blind eye to this type of maltreatment. People of the jury, hopefully you will have a brave advocate such as Dr. Trader when you are callously injured by a trusted physician like Dr. Jackson. He did not know, or did not follow, this basic tenant of treating heart attacks.

"Dr. Trader risks being spurned by the smug, clubby physician culture to do the right thing. Pray that you would have such an advocate. Think about this tonight."

◧   ◧   ◧

I drove to Noah's house. It was thirty-five degrees and raining. I felt like ducking to keep from hitting my head on the low clouds. No wonder everyone in Oregon walks around with heads down during winter.

Noah looked terrible. His normally shining face looked dim, as if the lamp inside had run out of kerosene.

He pulled off his tie and flung it to the floor. He went to the refrigerator and pulled out two beers, "One for me, and the other for me."

I asked, "Where's Suzie?"

"Her sister's wedding is this week. They're all having fun in San Diego and I'm being drawn and quartered." He cracked a beer, "I'm not going to drink much, but a beer or two might help me relax. I have to endure the torture again tomorrow." He told me the details of the trial.

I said, "What does your lawyer think?"

"I met with Reggie a few minutes ago. He said multiple jurors seemed to agree with what was said about me. He noticed at least four of them nodding in agreement with Dr. Dorcas, and then stealing harsh glances at me. He thought that the plaintiffs lawyers had sprung a masterful trap; have Franklin be the thoughtful doctor, and Dr. Dorcas be the bad cop who reinforces what Franklin said.

"They knew Reggie could discredit Dorcas, but Dorcas enforced and repeated the respectable opinion offered by the esteemed Dr. Franklin Trader.

"Reggie said he was worried; things weren't going as well as he'd hoped."

I said, unconvincingly, "I'm sure it'll be fine." A hollow platitude, I felt like a dork as soon as the words left my mouth. I might as well have said, "Smile and the whole world smiles with you!"

He said, "Why did I choose emergency medicine? I could've been a businessman like my father. He never got sued, nor did any of his friends. I could've been a coach, an airline pilot, an astronaut, anything but this. Even after I made the mistake of medical school, I could've been a radiologist or a dermatologist; they never get sued.

"Why did I spend years of my life for this? One patient out of thousands has a bad outcome and all of my earthly belongings and my reputation are imperiled. One patient.

"Twelve people—none of them with medical training—will decide if I should've given clot busting drugs. How's that a jury of my peers? Those twelve people will determine whether I should be permanently bankrupted. If I lose this case, I'll lose my house, any chance of paying for potential children's college, any chance of retiring before age one hundred. I won't be able to get a credit card with that kind of debt."

He brought his beer up to his taut face.

He continued, "Mr. Jerome Bristol: I saved his life and this is the thanks I get? He was dying. He was going toward the light and I shocked him back to earth. He can't play golf anymore after chain-smoking his entire life and he wants to blame me? He wants to put me into permanent debt?"

He paused, drained his first beer then continued, "Franklin Trader: could there be a more despicable human on the planet? Reggie told me that Franklin knew Mr. Bristol from playing golf at the Briarwood County Club. He probably encouraged Mr. Bristol to sue. A lawsuit was born. The fact that he knew Mr. Bristol almost certainly had something to do with his willingness to testify.

"Franklin will be rewarded handsomely. Most doctors who testify earn at least three times our normal hourly wage.

"I'm fairly certain the reason I'm being sued is the intervention of Franklin Trader." He cracked a second beer and took a long pull.

I said, "He's flaunting all convention; doctors who testify in weak cases like this are seen as Benedict Arnolds. Most of us fear lawsuits more than death. How can we plan for our future when one patient can take it all away? Either Franklin doesn't realize what he's doing, or he doesn't care. Or he knows what he's doing and he thinks he's doing the right thing by standing up for justice."

Noah said, "Or he knows precisely what he is doing; he is trying to murder me in broad daylight."

I had a feeling it was the last scenario. Franklin's ego was a ravenous beast. His ego had been fed at each level of victory, when he got into Yale, med school, and residency. The beast grew and needed more. The only way to satisfy the beast was to win, to kill, to drink the blood from the skull of your enemies.

He went to the fridge for another beer or three. He kept drinking. We sat silently.

Noah broke the silence, "Why should I continue to be a doctor? To help mankind? To help hurting people? To heal the sick?

"Who am I, Gandhi or Mother Teresa? I'm pretty good with a hammer. Maybe I could do construction work.

"I've been miserable and depressed. I plan to turn my life around; now I can be depressed and miserable." He smiled grimly at the joke. Neither of us laughed.

He opened a fifth beer.

I said, "I'm really, really sorry. Call me when you get out of the courtroom tomorrow." I hugged him and then drove home.

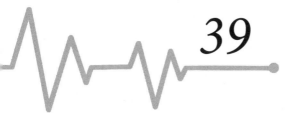

39

The next morning, Noah called me during a break, "What was I thinking? I'm hung over during the trial. I haven't gotten that drunk in years.

"This morning, I lay in bed for an hour and a half, with waves of nausea. I got up, showered, shaved, and put my other tie on, hangman's knot.

"I'm such an idiot. Maybe I should become a skid row alcoholic, since I'm looking for a new career. I can go bother Dr. Franklin Trader in his ER and hopefully puke on him."

I said, "Are you still nauseated? I could bring you some Zofran."

"I feel a little better since I've decided to quit medicine. Even if I lose the trial, they'll never collect since I won't make any money. Ha! Take that!"

He laughed, the first time I had heard him laugh in weeks. But it wasn't a happy laugh; it was a cackle, like the laugh of a psycho in a straitjacket.

"To answer your question, I'm nauseated but there ain't no medicine that will help me. I'm nauseated from drinking, nauseated from the stress, and nauseated from what I'm hearing: nausea, nausea everywhere. At one point this morning, I actually thought I was about to vomit.

"That would have been the lowest point of my existence, spewing beer and bile all over the courtroom with Franklin gazing in amusement. I could imagine it: my mouth flying open and my tormented soul projectile escaping from this wretched vessel holding it, before being mopped up by the courthouse janitor."

⊞　　⊞　⊞

I said, "Do you want to go get dinner or something?"

He said, "No, I'm mired in self-loathing and misery. I feel truly horrible, almost like I have the flu. I had the worst night of drunken sleep last night and the most miserable day of my life.

"I'm going to sleep early to sleep as long as possible."

That night, I couldn't sleep. I felt so sorry for Noah. My mind was racing and thoughts were firing through my head, none of them nice—loathing of Franklin, pity for Noah, regret at my career choice, disgust for Franklin, anxiety of mistakes, fear of lawsuits, abhorrence of Franklin.

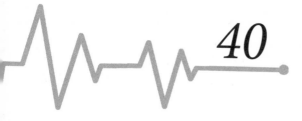

40

I sat with Noah in a diner. I ate and he poked at his eggs. He said, "I'm worried about my sanity. This trial opened a door between the sane and insane."

I said, "Well, close it quick."

Ignoring me, he said, "I've decided there's no way I'm going to continue to be an ER doctor; this stuff is bad for the soul. A man isn't made to endure bizarre hours of work, combined with torn and ripped bodies, mixed with blame and shame. I don't need it."

I smiled sadly.

He looked at his watch and said, "I gotta go. It's time for me to report to my personal torture chamber. I wonder if they will strap me on the rack, or tie me to a post and whip me with a cat-o-nine-tails. The judge seemed like a hooded torturer in his dark robes. I half expected him to bang his gavel and say, 'Please strip Dr. Jackson naked and attach electrical cables.'"

◻ ◻ ◻

After the initial proceedings, Dr. Hans Maier took the podium. He was the final witness. Reggie began, "Dr. Maier, what's your professional background?"

Dr. Maier responded, "I've been an emergency physician since 1972. In 1980, I was recruited to OHSU in Portland and became a Full Professor and Director of the Emergency Department. I stepped down in 1990 to spend more time teaching and interacting with the residents; I've been the Residency Director since 1997. I've published over one hundred academic articles. I was President of the American Academy of Emergency Physicians from 1995 to 2000. I've edited several academic textbooks."

A spark of hope.

Reggie continued, "What do you think of the care provided by Dr. Noah Jackson in this case?"

Dr. Maier answered, "As his teacher, I say with pride that he handled the case as I would've. He did things as quickly as possible and dealt with the case expertly. He shocked Mr. Bristol back to life and administered six stabilizing medicines. He obtained expert backup. He consulted the Cardiologist and they made a decision based on maximum patient benefit."

Reggie asked, "What do you think about the testimony provided by Drs. Trader and Dorcas?"

Dr. Maier said, "I don't know Dr. Dorcas, but I've heard him testify before. I'm not surprised.

"I am, however, flabbergasted by Dr. Franklin Trader's testimony. Having been his teacher, I cannot believe that he'd simplify the care for a complex heart attack down to a simple one-page flow chart in a textbook. That's like showing how to build an airplane on a single page."

Franklin probably cared deeply what Dr. Maier thought of him. To be criticized publicly was likely not anticipated when he signed on for this adventure. He probably thought Noah was the only person he would know at the trial, and Noah was the only one who would be publicly criticized. He had no way of knowing that he would be going head to head with Dr. Maier. Dr. Maier commands respect; he is to our residency as the Pope is to Catholics.

Noah's spark was fanned into a small flame.

Dr. Maier continued, "Dr. Jackson and the cardiologist took a more nuanced view of treatment than a one page flow chart would suggest. Of course they would! A cardiologist specializes in treating heart problems. That's all they do; they are highly sub-specialized in cardiac care.

"Dr. Trader thinks Dr. Jackson should have overruled the cardiologist and done what he wanted? Would Dr. Trader think it wise if a med student did what he thought best, rather than listen to a faculty doctor? The person with the most training has the final word in a case like this. The cardiologist would defer to Dr. Jackson in treating a car accident victim.

"I couldn't believe Dr. Trader would fault checking multiple EKGs on this patient. That's standard teaching: the more EKGs in a patient like this, the more information to make a decision.

"I'm deeply disappointed in Dr. Trader and I am very proud of the treatment rendered by Dr. Jackson. I'm saddened that Mr. Bristol was injured. I wish the cath lab had been available the night of his heart attack. Given the circumstances, there's nothing more Dr. Jackson could have done."

Noah's flame was stoked into a fire.

For cross-examination, Mr. Bristol's lawyer held up the textbook he had used the day before. "Dr. Maier, do you think this is an authoritative textbook?"

"That's an excellent textbook."

"Why doesn't this book say transferring a heart attack to another hospital is an option? There are two options: cath versus immediate CB treatment. Are you contradicting the primary textbook in your field?"

Dr. Maier moved in for the kill, "I'm glad you brought that up. That textbook is Goldfrank's Principles of Emergency Medicine, correct? Can you open it to page two? Whose photo do you see there?"

The lawyer flipped it open. He did not say anything.

Dr. Maier continued, "That's my photo. I'm one of the primary editors of that textbook."

Several jurors laughed out loud. Noah summoned all of his self-control not to join them.

He continued, "I should explain to the jury: while a textbook is a good source of information, medicine is a rapidly changing field. The information in a brand new textbook is several years old by the time it hits the bookstores. It's not like a history textbook with minor revisions done with each edition. An up-to-date emergency doctor will glean information mostly from academic journals. Textbooks are typically for residents and med students.

"Several recent studies have shown that cardiac cath is far superior to CB treatment. The bulk of scientific evidence is moving away from CB treatment and toward caths due to lower complication rates and better long-term outcomes. The complications that can be seen with CB include bleeding into the brain. Not mild side effects: devastation.

"Dr. Jackson was acting as a well-read Emergency Doctor when he chose the plan of action for Mr. Bristol. Could the outcome have been better if he had gotten CB treatment? Possibly. Could it have been worse? Possibly. In fact, from a statistical viewpoint, the data suggests it would have been worse.

"If Dr. Trader had taken the time to read the first five pages of this textbook, he would've seen my editor's notes, explaining this basic principle.

"I was residency director for both of them. Dr. Jackson consistently—consistently—got excellent evaluations from the faculty. The best. He's a very careful, very thoughtful physician. I'd let him take care of my wife or my mother."

⊡　⊡　⊡

Noah called me. He said, "The trial's over. The jury is deliberating. This dingy room is driving me crazy. Two of the four fluorescent lights are dark; another is flickering. Water is dripping from a cheap sink like Chinese water torture. I'm about to jump out the window if they don't hurry up and decide this thing. Not knowing is excruciating."

"What do you think about it?"

"I still think I'll lose. I just hope it's not above my policy limits."

"What did Dr. Maier say?"

"He was awesome. He opened up with both barrels and let the hot lead fly. Check this out: Bristol's team used the textbook that Dr. Maier edited. He pointed it out and a few jurors laughed out loud."

"What did he say?"

"He asked them to look at the editor's photo. It was like something from a movie. He also said a one-page flow chart was a vast oversimplification of a complex disease."

"Did he say anything about Franklin?"

"Yeah, he unloaded on him, two shells point blank to the chest. In the words of NWA, 'When I got a sawed off, bodies are hauled off.'"

"The rapping doctor. You must be feeling better."

"Not really. I feel good about the beating Dr. Maier gave Franklin. Frankie looked like someone who had been kicked in the gut and was trying to act like it didn't hurt."

I laughed, "When do you find out the verdict?"

"I don't know. Whenever they decide. I'm prepared for the worst. I'm expecting the worst."

I searched for something encouraging.

He said, "I need to go. I want to call Suzie. I'll call you when I find out."

I felt sick. My nerves flailed like I'd drunk ten cups of coffee. I pondered everything. The things Noah said the night he was drunk bothered me, deeply. His reasons for wanting to quit medicine were some of the same concerns I had felt, since early residency. The concerns I had tried to minimize, tried to bury.

The weird hours are not healthy. Grim devastation and death takes a toll. A father jumping off a parking garage sticks like hot tar flung from a stick.

We want to be, need to be, perfect and we are not. Errors are inevitable and the stakes are high. We judge ourselves harshly, and we feel harshly judged. We are escorting wheelchairs across an icy lake.

From a patient's perspective, it doesn't matter if a mistake was the only mistake made in a decade. If they are injured, perhaps severely, by a medical error, they have every right to want justice and compensation.

I had to do something to clear my mind. I put on my running shoes and stepped outside, into the cool rain. Six p.m.: the city was winding down, and winding up.

I started to run. I ran down the damp neighborhood street and rounded a corner. I picked up speed. An ambulance sped past, the lights on. I ran harder. I ducked around umbrellas. I jumped a puddle.

My lungs ached. My heart battered my sternum. I ran past a drunk teenager on a park bench.

I ran from anxiety. I ran from fear.

I kept running, even harder. I was exhausted, but could not stop. My feet hammered the pavement. I was trying to kill something, to kill the dread and the turmoil. I was scared for Noah, but I was scared of something else. I was not sure why I was scared..

I ran like the Mississippi cops were chasing. I ran like a frightened man.

I jogged across the Hawthorne Bridge. I ran through downtown, weaving between business people. I crossed the Burnside Bridge, dodging homeless people. I cut through nice parks and run-down neighborhoods. I ran beside old churches and seedy strip joints. I just ran.

My lungs burned. I felt blisters, fluid filled on my toes. I ran for hours. I did not want to stop. I felt blisters rupture. Like a cutter, the pain distracted me from my real affliction.

Finally, I could not go on. I limped back to my house. I sat on the steps in front of the house, wet with sweaty rain and dripping with nerves.

I pondered.

◘ ◘ ◘

Missy came to the door. She said, "Noah's called twice on your phone. Call him back!"

I dialed the phone.

Noah said, "The jury decided in our favor. They deliberated for less than two hours. Reggie estimated that Mr. Bristol's law firm lost several hundred thousand dollars litigating the case."

I laughed out loud, "Wow. That's killer!" I flashed thumbs up to Missy and she did a little cheerleader move.

Noah said, "I saw Dr. Maier outside the courtroom after the trial. I rushed over to thank him. He was characteristically humble and seemed awkward at my praises. Listen to this! He said, 'I almost never speak ill of graduates from our program but Franklin committed malpractice according to the standards of the American Medical Association. He was quite dishonest about numerous things. If we sent a copy of his testimony to the AMA, he'd be severely reprimanded. He'd likely be placed on a list of physicians the AMA considers fraudulent witnesses. If they do that, it would open a door to obtain justice for this travesty.

"'If the AMA considers him a fraudulent witness, his partners at St. Paul's could terminate his employment. He's under a two-year trial period and this is probably enough to get him fired. He'd have a very hard time finding employment after that.'"

I said, "Unbelievable."

"Yeah, I know. Dr. Maier said that he knows the director at St. Paul's; he helped Franklin get his job. He said, 'I'm not going to call him about this, but if he calls me, I won't hold back.' He winked at me when he said it."

I said, "Dude! That's great! Let's go celebrate! We could have a bonfire and burn Frankie in effigy!"

"Maybe another night. I don't feel like celebrating; I feel like a survivor of a violent assault. I can't drink anything. I can't stand the sight of the beer; I took all the beer out of my fridge yesterday."

"What're you going to do about Dr. Maier's suggestion?"

"I already called the courthouse and asked for a CD copy of Franklin's testimony. They said it'd be mailed to my house within a week."

I laughed with glee, "Ha! Take that Dr. Traitor! He who laughs last, laughs best."

"I guess. I don't have the energy for any more right now. I want to focus my thoughts and think rationally. I want to deal with the incident and put it to rest. Close the chapter and move on.

"I don't want to let this incident sour me on medicine or people. That's not how I was raised. I don't want to be a bitter person. To be able to help others in their time of need is an incredible privilege and honor."

I never knew what to expect from him.

He waxed on philosophically, "I feel like there are four ways most people waste much of their energy and therefore waste their lives: regretting the past, futile worry about the future, thinking negative thoughts about others, and worrying about other people thinking poorly of them.

"I've failed on all four fronts. I'm embarrassed at how sorry I've been feeling for myself.

"At least I can still golf."

⊡   ⊡   ⊡

The backbone of the case had been Franklin Trader and his willingness to testify against a colleague.

The backbone had been snapped in half when it was struck head on by a charging rhino: Dr. Hans Maier. Vertebrae splintered and collapsed, crushed under the weight of a mightier beast.

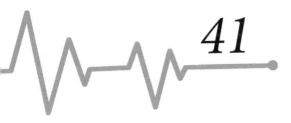

41

In the weeks after the trial, I felt like a dirty cloud had blown away, allowing light. I was relieved of the burden of angst I had been carrying. Nothing had really changed but my attitude, but it made a huge difference.

My partners knew Noah and Franklin since both were residents at Brookwood. All were aghast and angry at Franklin's dishonest testimony. I couldn't wait for Noah to fire off letters to the AMA and St Paul's to make Franklin pay. I wanted him to do it yesterday. Punish that Traitor.

I had a string of entertaining shifts and work was fun again. Patients seemed like friends instead of adversaries.

My job—my calling—deals with injury and death. A platoon sergeant would love to keep all his troops alive, but he cannot, not during war. If he cannot handle losing some, he should not have accepted the job. If I could not handle the responsibility and the pressures, then I should not have become an emergency physician. I could handle it—I was built for it. I didn't choose emergency medicine; it chose me. All my whining and perseveration about stress, drama, and perfection seemed silly.

I remembered the rafting trip my intern year. I had a sense of belonging like I had never felt before. I found my tribe, my people. As time passed, this has proven true. I know of no other occupation where the majority of social contacts and friendships come from the same profession. Over half of my friends are ER doctors. Our schedules, struggles, interests, and personalities are similar. We understand each other.

A few months after the trial, I was back at work and in my groove. I was halfway through a typical shift. I had a few patients to discharge and a few in the rack to see. I was working with Nate: Fruit-Of-The-Loom-Man, Defender of the Justice and Yuppies.

A nurse yelled, "Brent, we need you in here!" She was walking back with a mother and a panting, terrified child. I rushed over. I could see the child was in trouble, big trouble.

I knew at first glace she had epiglottitis—the murderer of children.

She was in the sniffing position, craning her chin forward with both hands on her knees. She found this position because her airway was closing. Swallowing was excruciatingly painful, so she drooled. Her face commingled pain and fright.

I said, "Let's give her oxygen and a breathing treatment." I quietly told a nurse, "Set up for intubation and a surgical airway. She needs IV rocephin, one gram."

Her mother quavered, "She's suffocating."

I said, "You're in a safe place. How long has she been sick?"

"She had a high fever when she went to bed and said her throat was owie. She woke me up with noisy breathing and drooling. I saw the look on her face and rushed her here. She looks like she can barely breathe!"

Childhood epiglottitis is the strangler of children, like a snake in the crib. Franklin ridiculed me during residency for missing a case of adult epiglottitis, but no one would miss this. The little one was working very hard to suck air into her body. Everyone who saw her shared her agonizing fear, especially her mother.

And me.

Epiglottitis is a bacterial infection of the epiglottis: the flap that protects the airway during swallowing. The HIB vaccine for children has almost eradicated the disease, a public heath success and a huge relief to ER doctors. Epiglottitis was probably the most feared disease of my residency.

It was fearsome because a healthy child is at risk of dying in front of your eyes. The aggressive bacteria cause rapid swelling of the epiglottis. The child is strangled from the inside—a malevolent serpent coiled and crushing the throat.

I led her mother to the side and said softly, "She has an infection causing swelling in her throat. She'll need a breathing tube, but for now, we should try to keep her calm. We aren't going to do anything until she goes to the operating room. We should be quiet and calming because that will help her survive this."

Her mother was a timid, kind-appearing woman, like a librarian. She nodded tearfully and returned to her daughter, "It's O.K., baby. It's O.K. The doctors are going to help you."

Her name was Madison and she had three candles on her last birthday cake. Madison's brow was furrowed with confusion and pain. Tears ran silently down her soft cheeks. Her mother soothingly rubbed her back, quickly wiping her own tears.

I wanted to keep Madison calm because she was breathing through a tiny hole—like being restrained under deep water and struggling to breathe through a long drinking straw. If she panicked, the harder it would be to suck air through a cocktail straw. The smaller the hole, the more panic she would feel. The more she labored, the more likely the hole would close: completely and fatally.

Try explaining that to a 3-year-old.

I put out a stat page to the throat surgeon and the anesthesiologist. I said, "I have a 3-year-old with epiglottis." They each said, "I'm on my way." They were the two shortest conversations with consultants, ever.

The plan was to take her to the operating room where she could be intubated in the most controlled environment. If the anesthesiologist couldn't pass the tube due to swelling, the surgeon would cut a hole in Madison's neck to place an airway below the stranglehold.

We awaited their arrival. I felt like a silent sentry, standing guard but doing nothing. Madison and her mother both oozed fear: panic and hysteria flowing like lava beneath a thin veneer of calm, like crust about to collapse.

As Madison's nose flared and panic flared, her mother's wet eyes pled. Her eyes spoke, "Please, save my little girl."

To sit on my hands and wait was torment. I felt like someone watching the execution of an innocent family member. Each moment that passed, the snake constricted.

She breathed harder, seeming to sense her mother's panic. Madison's strawberry blonde hair hung in sweaty strands. My nerves shimmered like lightening on a lake.

We waited.

What's taking them so long? Where are the freaking anesthesiologist and the surgeon? I looked at the clock and it had been ten minutes. The expectation for arrival is thirty.

Madison's breathing slowed, and she looked sleepy. Her oxygen level dropped. Her head began to nod, a slow drift down and then a groggy jerk. I didn't want to alarm her mother, but it was an ominous sign.

There were a couple of possibilities: she could be past the point of exhaustion. Asthmatics tire out, but they usually have been working to breathe for hours; Madison had only labored for about an hour. More likely she was sleepy because she was not ridding her body of carbon dioxide; she was in respiratory failure. The carbon dioxide in her body was not leaving since the hole was too small. Carbon dioxide was accumulating in her blood, causing sleepiness. Causing death.

Her head drifted down and stayed down. She slumped sideways. Her eyes closed in sleep. Endless sleep.

I had to act. She needed to be intubated. I was on my own.

I hate intubating children for multiple reasons. A child's airway is obviously smaller but also anatomically different. We intubate children infrequently and even the most skilled ER doctor is a novice.

I said, "We have to intubate her. We can't wait any longer."

No one in the room knew the risk of what I had to do. The nurses did not know the likelihood of failure. Madison's mother was probably relieved that I was doing something.

Only I knew the terrible odds of this last ditch effort—the reason we wait to intubate in the operating room. Waiting had backfired: the worst-case scenario. We had waited until her airway was practically closed. By stalling, I made my task much more difficult and worsened her chance of survival.

Madison was nearly dead. I was the only thing between her and the murderous constrictor.

I did not want this. I wanted the anesthesiologist or the surgeon to take her to the Operating Room. They should do it. I was not qualified.

The biggest danger with intubating a child with epiglottitis is that touching the epiglottis with the tube will often cause total occlusion. I was going to get one shot. If I failed the epiglottis would snap shut like reptilian jaws.

If I failed the intubation, which seemed likely, I would have to do a surgical airway. It would be incredibly difficult as Madison had a short neck and the landmarks were difficult to find.

I had never performed a surgical airway on a child.

Never. As in *never*.

The hardest part of being an ER doctor is when the demands of the job do not fit the level of skill or training. I might need to do a complex procedure I had never done to keep Madison alive.

I would be puncturing a short beautiful neck with a scalpel, hoping and praying I was stabbing the right place. If I missed, she would never wake up.

She would never ride her big wheel, never eat ice cream, and never ask for a bedtime story again. Her last moments on earth would be her worst: being pierced by a frightened doctor.

The nurse nodded that she was ready. I said, "Give her one milligram of vecc and one of versed." The nurse gave the medicine.

One minute later, she was paralyzed and not breathing on her own. Time for battle—me against the snake.

Ready or not.

I dropped her head down and I scooped her tongue out of the way with the laryngoscope. I saw the swollen hot epiglottis, angry with pus and venom. I positioned the tube and prepared to push it through—an attempt to shove a sword into the mouth of a giant viper. I carefully aligned the tube to the center. My soul trembled.

I pushed it in. The epiglottis bit down, but I was already in.

I was in.

The tube slid through. I saw the fury of the beast with its mouth forced open.

Madison was intubated. The tube would resist all attempts of the enraged epiglottis to close, to deny entry of cool air past its poisonous fangs. It had no choice but to be held open, in an open position of vulnerability, sucking on a plastic tube, until the snake loosened his grip and fell away.

I removed my gloves, wiped my brow, and said to her mother, "She's intubated. She'll be OK. We'll admit her to the Pediatric Intensive Care Unit and she'll be treated with IV antibiotics. She'll probably be intubated for a few days, but she should recover fully." Her mother burst into tears and collapsed shaking into a chair. The nurse hugged her shoulders as she heaved.

I called the ICU doctor and arranged transfer to a children's hospital. Twenty minutes later, the transport team arrived and whisked her away.

My knee quaked.

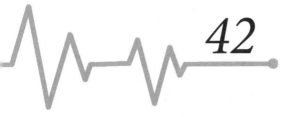

42

I was climbing Mount Hood with Noah. We hiked in the dark so we could reach the summit at daybreak; it's easier and safer to climb at night when the ice and snow are firm. We were roped together and he led as we began the steep ascent to the summit. We swung our ice axes into the hard snow with each step. My legs burned, and each breath visibly floated from our mouths like steam, similar to the steam that escaped from the volcano beneath our heavy boots. The sulfuric odor became pungent the higher we climbed.

Our headlamps illuminated the path. We hiked past the terrifying beautiful blue ice of exposed glacier, a gaping maw. The steep drop into the glacier meant a misstep could drop us both into the heart of the mountain: forever at one with the frozen volcano and the many souls who found their final rest there.

I broke the silence, "Did I tell you about the little girl with epiglottitis I intubated?"

"Really? Holy Saint Peter in Heaven! Why'd you intubate her?"

"I couldn't wait. She passed out in the ER."

"How'd she do?"

"She was fine. It was a tight fit squeezing the tube in. I was clenched."

"I bet you were. I hope I never have to do that. Thank God for the HIB vaccine; that disease has almost vanished. How'd she do?"

"Fine. She went home a week later. She'll live to have four candles on her cake. I was so alive after that shift, like I'd sacked the quarterback on fourth and goal. I'm feeling the love for the job again. I was pretty fried, between the drama of residency and your trial. I had second thoughts."

"You're telling me. I honestly thought I was done during the trial, no joke. I don't know what I would've done if we lost. I'm scared to think. It's weird to make a career choice based on an arbitrary jury's decision."

"It's weird that a jury's decision is arbitrary."

We hiked on. I had a question I really wanted to ask, but I did not want to ruin his mood.

Our breathing became more labored the higher we went. Our headlamps sliced through the night like searchlights. The moonlit snow radiated. Snow-covered rocks haunted the peak, ghosts. We pushed for the summit, climbing an almost vertical wall of ice, rock, and snow.

The spikes of his crampons were a few feet above my head as he kicked toeholds. My axe struck rock and clanged loudly in the silence. I swung again and it sunk satisfyingly into firm snow.

Near the top, I couldn't resist. I asked, "What happened with Frankie Boy?" I had not brought him up since the trial, as Noah seemed done with the topic. I was hoping he had put the fiery fury of vengeance into motion.

He said, "That's funny you asked. This week I was cleaning out my desk. I found the transcript of Franklin's testimony in a stamped envelope to the American Medical Association's Ethics Committee. Another letter was addressed to the director at St Paul's Hospital. I heard that his partners weren't happy with the negative publicity, and let him know."

I laughed, "I bet they were less than thrilled. Time to pay, Judas-Brutus."

He struggled to gain purchase with his ice axe then spoke, "He's really a person I should pity, not hate. That guy will never succeed enough to be happy. Anyone who needs fame, fortune, looks, prestige, athletic ability, or that new leather sofa to be happy—will never be happy."

"That's true, but we don't want him to be happy. The thought of him makes me want to chew glass."

He was silent for a few steps; the altitude made each word a chore. He said, "Franklin's background and personality created a deep-seated insecurity. Maybe his parents were overbearing, or he got picked on." He took a few hard breaths, and continued, "He has an unhealthy ego that's quick to brag, defend, or attack. His inner dragon is more of a scared child, I suspect.

"I've been wallowing in mud; the trial was such a thorn in my side. I wasted so much time with my inability to rise above. I allowed my ego to drag me into a dark, dark place. I'm done with that.

"I tore the letters into pieces. I trashed it. It was so cathartic to step away."

I said, "Wow. I'd want to make him pay. If Dr. Maier talks with his director, Franklin could get fired. Don't you think he should pay?"

He said, "Believe me, I know what you're saying, and part of me aches for revenge. But, in some ways, he has paid. Dr. Maier smacked him down, and the entire ER community knows. He won't do it again.

"Hate is drinking poison and waiting for him to die. I don't want that. He'll never know I spared him, but I don't care. I forgive him."

I pondered. We climbed a few more minutes until we reached the summit. I felt something thaw inside.

We were alone, on the top of the world. The dawn approached, the darkness draining away. Moments later, the sun split the horizon, brilliant and warm on my face. The snow turned from dusky gray to white, white as a bridal gown.

I smiled. It was a new day.

AFTERWORD

⊡   ⊡   ⊡

These events happened years ago, so minor details are subject to the failings of my memory. I verified as many facts as possible. I interviewed Noah's lawyer and the doctors involved in these cases. I reviewed the transcript of Noah's court case. I altered names to protect privacy, both of patients and friends. I've worked at more than one hospital in Portland, lumped together as Brookwood. The original dialogue and exact words spoken have long faded, but I attempted to stay true to the spirit of those conversations. Minor points have been changed to hide identifiers and to help with the flow of the book. Some of the stories have been simplified, but not exaggerated: the truth is bizarre enough. I don't think my experience is exceptional; any of my partners could have written this book.

The timing is not completely accurate. I remember more details and the exact timing of events and patients that had a big impact on me. For example, I saw Myron shortly after starting at Brookwood, and Phillip jumped before the trial, but other stories are randomly placed. I wove interesting cases from different shifts to create a sense of moving between patients. The exception is chapter thirty-five; I saw all of those patients on the same Full Moon Night.

Ricky is the only major character I've lost contact with. A few of the stories attributed to him came from different paramedics. Ricky's story about Freakdog was presented at a medical conference. I created those characters' personal details.

When I discussed Crank the Clown with Jordie, he said, "I haven't told many people that story because I'm worried they'll think I'm lying." Emergency medicine is stranger than fiction.

Last winter, Noah and I went on a guided backcountry skiing trip in the Canadian Rockies. We hiked in a single file line on the knife-edge of a steep ridge, our skis strapped to our backpacks. There were steep drops on both sides as we hiked above the slope that we planned to ski. Noah was next to me when we heard an ominous low boom: a gigantic avalanche slab broke five yards below us, carrying the slope we intended to ski over a five hundred foot cliff, like a waterfall of snow. If we had been on the slope when it went, we would have almost certainly arrived at Heaven's Gates wearing snow goggles.

Noah is one of the best friends I've ever had and we live on the same street. Missy and Suzie are friends, our sons play together.

And Noah still tries to beat me down the hill.

Check out the video made by Brent, Noah, Missy, Nate, Seth, Marge, and others, as they dramatize several scenes from Miracles and Mayhem.

If you like it, send it to your friends and family!

DocRockRussell.com

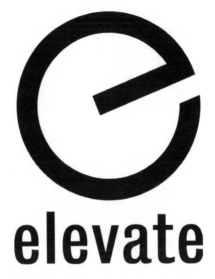

elevate

Strategic publishing empowering authors to strengthen their brand.

Visit Elevate for our latest offerings:

www.elevatepub.com